Good Nights

Good Nights

((*(*(*(*(*(*

How to Stop Sleep Deprivation, Overcome Insomnia, and Get the Sleep You Need

(

DR. GARY ZAMMIT

WITH JANE A. ZANCA

(

Produced by Alison Brown Cerier
Book Development, Inc.

**Andrews McMeel
Publishing**

Kansas City

A hardcover edition of this book was published in 1997 by Andrews McMeel Publishing.

The recommendations and information in this book are appropriate in most cases, but you should consult a personal physician or a sleep center for individual problems.

The names that appear in case studies and examples throughout this book have been changed.

Library of Congress Cataloging-in-Publication Data
Zammit, Gary K.
    Good nights : how to stop sleep deprivation, overcome insomnia, and get the sleep you need / Gary Zammit with Jane A. Zanca.
       p.   cm.
    Includes index.
    ISBN 0-8362-5275-6 (ppb)
      1. Sleep—Popular works. 2. Sleep disorders—Popular works. I. Zanca, Jane A. II. Title.
RA786.Z36 1997
616.8'498—dc21   96-47819
                                              CIP

Book design by Susan Hood.

* ☾ *

To Kristin
FOR THE DREAMS WE'VE
SHARED

— GKZ

To my father

— JAZ

Contents

Preface

My coauthor and I have written this book for the millions of people who suffer from sleep deprivation. It is our hope to provide important, practical information about sleep deprivation, insufficient sleep, and sleep disorders.

Perhaps it will be the stimulus for you to initiate a dialogue with your health provider regarding sleep, or it may result in a referral to a sleep-disorders center. However, the main focus of this book is to provide a step-by-step, self-help program for healthy sleep. This program has been used successfully by hundreds of people with sleep problems. Many have experienced significant improvements in their sleep, daytime functioning, and quality of life.

It is my hope that readers of this book can use the program with or without the guidance of a doctor. Although this book is not a replacement for medical care, in most cases it can be used effectively as a self-help remedy for sleep deprivation. The recommendations in this book are the same ones that I would give you if you were sitting with me in my office in Manhattan. I have every confidence that you, or someone you care about who uses this program, can expect results that are quite similar to those achieved by my patients here.

Your response to the program will vary with the nature of your sleep problem, its severity, and your determination and persistence. With time and reflection, though, you can develop a program tailored to your specific needs that will offer you the maximum likelihood of success—just as we would do in my office.

If sleep deprivation continues to be a problem after you have followed the program in this book, you may be suffering from a serious sleep disorder or have a problem that cannot be treated with conventional therapies. In these cases, I strongly suggest that you consult with your health provider or pursue treatment with a specialist at a sleep-disorders clinic.

It's a credit to the progress we've made in understanding sleep disorders that such centers exist. Twenty years ago, there were only a few sleep-disorders centers. The United States now has more than 888 board-certified sleep specialists and more than 310 sleep-disorders centers accredited by the American Sleep Disorders Association. Consultation with one of these professionals will enable you to obtain state-of-the-art diagnostic testing, as well as sophisticated drug and nondrug therapies for your sleep problem.

One such clinic is the Sleep Disorders Institute I founded and run. It is Manhattan's largest accredited sleep-disorders center and part of St. Luke's–Roosevelt Hospital Center, a teaching hospital of Columbia University College of Physicians and Surgeons. I am also an associate professor at Columbia, a clinical psychologist with more than eighteen years of experience in the field of sleep, and certified by the American Board of Sleep Medicine. I am a member of several national sleep committees and a former member of New York State's Governor's Task Force on the Impact of Fatigue on Driving.

I encourage you to take full advantage of my years of experience and those of other sleep specialists and hundreds of people who have suffered from sleep deprivation, all of which have gone into the preparation of this book. I believe that this program will provide you with a lifetime of good nights from which you will awaken refreshed and ready to begin each new day.

I would like to acknowledge the support of my mentors, Drs. Harold Zepelin, Thomas Roth, and Charles Pollak for the invaluable lessons that they have taught, and especially Dr. Sigurd Ackerman for allowing me the opportunity to work on this book. I would also like to thank my colleagues at the Sleep Disorders Institute, Drs. Stephen

Lund, Joseph Ghassibi, and Kathleen Rice; Ms. Vanessa Oritz, Ms. Eileen Rose, and Ms. Joan Hirschfeld; and the technical and research staff for providing a work environment that has enabled me to devote time to this project. I would like to thank Ms. Erlyn Depena for typing the manuscript. Finally, I would like to thank Ms. Alison Brown Cerier for developing the manuscript and editing the book and Ms. Jane Zanca for her collaboration in translating my scientific writing into a text that can be read, understood, and enjoyed by you.

Good Nights

* 1 *

Why You Need to Stop Sleep Deprivation

- Are there days when you feel you could fall asleep earlier, or stay in bed longer, if you let yourself?
- Do you sleep much later than usual on the weekends?
- Are you dragging around during the day? Do you need a good jolt or two of caffeine to feel truly awake?
- Are you fighting sleepiness in meetings, or when you sit down to watch a movie or TV show?
- Are people avoiding you because you're irritable, depressed, or not yourself? Are you saying things that you later realize you shouldn't have said?
- Are you feeling anxious?
- Are you having problems with mental tasks? How many times do you have to add or subtract columns in your checkbook to get them right? Are you making mistakes at work?
- Are people waving their arms and blowing their horns at you in the morning because your inattention is causing near accidents?
- Are you wearing out during physical tasks faster than you used to?
- Does it seem like you're picking up colds, viruses, and other unpleasant health problems at a higher rate than usual? Are you using up your sick days because you're "just not feeling well"?

If these questions make you feel uncomfortable and if you often answered yes, you are probably one of the millions of people suffering
from sleep deprivation. You may have insomnia—difficulty falling or
remaining asleep—but you may not. There are many other causes of
sleep deprivation too. Sleep deprivation is simply the condition of
not having as much restful sleep as you need.

WHAT CAUSES SLEEP DEPRIVATION?

For many people, the source of sleep deprivation is their own behavior and habits. We steal hours from our sleep time to work or play.
This habit has been growing ever stronger since the invention of the
electric light bulb made it easy to stay busy well into the night.

Among the first to buy into the advantages of this new invention
were industrialists, who quickly saw that it was more cost-effective to
sustain production than it was to start it at sunrise and stop it at sun-
set. To keep production lines moving, workers were soon expected
to report for extended work schedules, evening and night shifts, and
that peculiar twentieth-century torture, rotating shifts. Workers had
to restructure their sleep time, family activities, and recreational time.
Although many practices of the Industrial Revolution have gone by
the wayside, shift work is still with us. Of all full-time workers, 15.9
percent are shift workers. Now that we are entering the era of a global
economy, we are seeing new versions of shift work emerge to accommodate communication and commerce across international time zones.

Advances in technology now allow us to work and play around the
clock. We have continuous access to television, radio, telephone, fax,
and the World Wide Web. More and more businesses stay open twenty-
four hours for catalog orders, banking, or middle-of-the-night grocery shopping. More people telecommute from home, which provides
valuable flexibility but may mean that the long break for a trip to the
health club means finishing up work at midnight instead of sleeping.

While we are reaping flexibility and new opportunities from the
twenty-four-hour lifestyle, it's becoming more difficult for us to fill
our sleep needs. Over the past century, Americans have reduced their
average nightly total sleep time by more than 20 percent, or about
two hours a night!

While many people cheat themselves of sleep, others are cheated of the sleep they need by a sleep disorder. Insomnia, difficulty falling or staying asleep, is widespread. Sleep apnea, in which the sleeper must arouse or awaken to resume breathing, affects an astonishing eight million people in the United States. The current *International Classification of Sleep Disorders*, a handbook used by health professionals and scientists around the world to define the source of a sleep problem, identifies more than eighty disorders, each with distinctive signs and symptoms. These disorders afflict millions of us. According to recent reports forty million Americans are chronically ill with sleep disorders, and an additional twenty to thirty million experience intermittent sleep problems. This number is approximately 28 percent of our population! In a ripple effect, these people influence the lives of millions more.

In addition to sleep disorders, underlying medical or psychiatric illnesses often play a role, particularly for older people. For example, painful arthritis or enlarged prostate (which can cause a frequent urge to urinate) can disrupt sleep repeatedly, even when no other sleep disorders exist. Depression and anxiety also disrupt sleep.

Sleep deprivation can result from

- Your decision to do other things in the time that should be spent sleeping, even though you know the consequences
- Circumstances imposed on you, such as having to work shifts, hold two jobs, or care for a loved one who is seriously ill
- Not knowing how much time you should set aside for sleep
- A sleep disorder
- A medical or psychiatric condition that disrupts normal sleep patterns
- A combination of these causes

THE CONSEQUENCES OF SLEEP DEPRIVATION

Just because Americans are sleeping less than they used to does not mean they need less sleep. Sleep is the most basic human need. One can go longer without food and water, and certainly longer without sexual activity, than one can go without sleep.

What does sleep deprivation do to you and to others around you? Here are two excerpts from recent Congressional hearings held by the National Commission on Sleep Disorders Research.

> I was experiencing constant daytime drowsiness. I would fall into a deep sleep for short periods during meetings, conversations, and public functions. At times, I could awaken and make a very inappropriate comment, only to realize that I was commenting on a dream I had just experienced! My associates began to question my mental stability.

Like many who suffer from sleep deprivation, he failed to acknowledge the problem until it was so serious that it became visible to others. Another person who testified, a police officer for more than twelve years, first became aware of his sleep deprivation on the night he supervised the investigation of a violent physical assault:

> The graveyard shift has always been difficult for me—I could sleep only two or three hours a day. . . . The adrenaline surge such a [violent] scene might have provoked failed me entirely due to the overpowering effects of sleep exhaustion. I found myself fighting to stay awake during interviews, scene investigation, and arrest. . . . I found out later that some of the decisions I did make were inappropriate. . . . At a sleep center, doctors found that my body clock had never adapted to the graveyard shift, even after months of working on it.

Testimonials like these are common. I could recount hundreds more, some reporting minor inconveniences, others a significant impact on well-being and health.

Sleepiness

As in both the cases above, the most prominent sign of sleep deprivation is sleepiness. The fifty-dollar word for sleepiness is hypersomnolence (hyper = excessive, somnolent = sleep-inducing). Dr. Wilse Webb, one of the founding fathers of sleep science, once commented with good humor, "After years of studying sleep, one of the sure things known about sleep deprivation is that it makes you sleepy."

Undoubtedly, you know from your own experience that sleepiness will follow just one night of very little sleep. You may not realize that the same effects can come from small amounts of lost sleep, adding up over weeks and months.

Sleep deprivation can also occur when you were in bed for the right number of hours, and went to sleep and rose at normal times, but your sleep was disrupted or fragmented by a sleep disorder or medical problem. For example, periodic limb movement disorder causes muscle spasms that disrupt sleep. Another condition, sleep apnea, disrupts sleep even more dramatically—the sleeper stops breathing and must arouse or awaken to begin breathing again! For either condition, the person is usually unaware that he or she has been waking up many times during the night, but a haggard appearance and complaints of fatigue and irritability provide strong evidence that something is wrong.

The intensity of hypersomnolence depends on the amount of needed sleep that's been lost, the time of day, what's going on around you, and your age. A mild problem may be experienced as a slight difficulty staying alert or wakeful when involved in quiet or boring activities. You may catch yourself nodding off with a book in your lap or falling asleep at a committee meeting. Just about everyone has experienced this. If you often fall asleep in front of the television in the evening, the problem isn't that the show is boring, but that you're short on sleep.

Severe hypersomnolence can interfere with the ability to sustain involvement in any task, no matter how stimulating, and the person may fall asleep at inappropriate times. It's at this level of hypersomnolence that a Georgia school bus driver with a full load of active, noisy children on a busy street fell asleep.

If you try to deprive yourself of sleep for extended periods, your brain will take over, producing profound sleepiness or an overwhelming urge to sleep. Even when artificial means are used to keep a severely sleep-deprived person awake, the brain begins to show signs of "microsleeps," brief periods when the brain is fast asleep in a person who appears outwardly to be awake.

Psychological Effects

Sleep deprivation can dramatically alter one's emotional state. After extreme and prolonged sleep deprivation, people have been known to do things that under more normal conditions they would never do. In severe cases, they become aggressive or suspicious. And there have been reports of misperceptions, illusions, and hallucinations.

Even a small degree of sleep deprivation can result in depression, anxiety, or irritability. If the sleep deprivation persists night after night (whether due to a medical problem like sleep apnea or just to insufficient sleep), these emotional and personality changes go on day after day. Some people who are sleep deprived seek psychiatric care for their emotional problems, when the root of the problem is sleep deprivation.

Physical and Mental Effects

Interestingly, a person who is chronically sleep deprived may perform physical or mental tasks poorly at one time, but feel alert and perform well at another. Nevertheless, as sleep deprivation accumulates, hypersomnolence increases in general. Just about everyone who has stayed up through the night to study, work, or party can attest to feeling fatigued, sleepy, and less able to perform tasks, even simple ones.

It makes sense intuitively that sleep deprivation impairs performance, but what exactly happens? Studies have shown that even prolonged sleep deprivation does not impair *physical* functions dramatically. In studies in which the person was kept up continuously for thirty to seventy-two hours, heart, circulatory, or lung responses to exercise, aerobic capability, and muscle strength were not affected. However, sleep deprivation does decrease endurance, the amount of time that a person can exercise before becoming exhausted. It is likely that just about any physical feat achieved in a nondeprived state can be achieved in a sleep-deprived state—but not for quite as long. When might this condition matter? How about when you're being dragged away from shore by surf, and the lifeguard dashing into the water to save you has been up all night partying?

Mental performance is another matter. One of the earliest studies of the effects of sleep deprivation on mental performance was performed in the late ninteenth century at the Iowa University Psychological Laboratory. Drs. Patrick and Gilbert conducted an experiment in which Dr. Gilbert, then a twenty-eight-year-old "normal sleeper," remained awake for ninety hours, almost four full days. During the experiment the investigators discovered something very important: The

level of alertness fluctuated throughout the period of sleep deprivation. Sometimes Dr. Gilbert's alertness was normal or near normal,
and at other times it was obviously impaired. Sleepiness impaired alertness but could be overcome at certain times.

The findings of Patrick and Gilbert set the stage for twentieth-
century scientists' approach to the study of sleep deprivation. Several
studies, many conducted at the Walter Reed Army Institute of Research in Washington, D.C., in the 1950s and 1960s and many conducted much later, showed that extended sleep deprivation impaired
performance on tests of reaction time, vigilance, and memory. The
effects are greatest when a task is prolonged, boring, monotonous, or
complex. For example, one study showed that a person who can persist at a monotonous task without failure for ten minutes under normal conditions will be able to continue the task for only seven minutes
after one night of sleep deprivation and for only three minutes after
two nights of sleep deprivation.

These findings can be applied to real-life situations that are far removed from the laboratory. Sleep-deprived people may find that their
performance is impaired when they have to respond to a traffic light,
a prompt from a computer, or a business colleague's question. They
may have trouble remembering simple items like a grocery list or telephone number.

Yet a sleep-deprived person may be able to perform temporarily at
the usual level, as Dr. William Dement discovered more than 30 years
ago. A world-renowned sleep researcher from Stanford University,
Dr. Dement studied a seventeen-year-old boy named Randy Gard-
ner. Randy met Dr. Dement while completing a grueling 264-hour
vigil for a high school science fair project. Randy eventually achieved
his goal, establishing the world's record for prolonged wakefulness:
eleven days! In the middle of the last night of the vigil, Dr. Dement
and Randy spent several hours in a penny arcade, playing about one
hundred games on a baseball machine. Randy won every game, demon-
strating that neither his cognitive abilities nor his psychomotor functions were impaired.

*Unfortunately, the fact that the impairments can occasionally be overcome may
give us the false sense that we can defend against or control the effects of sleep deprivation.* This belief worsens the risk, especially when sleep-deprived
people are involved in potentially hazardous activities. It would be

interesting to know who drove home—Dr. Dement or Randy? Which one would you have taken a ride with?

Hormones and Sleep

Hormones are chemicals, produced by the body's glands, that control the body's functions. When you are in danger, adrenaline, produced by the adrenal glands, gets your heart pounding and your feet moving. Other hormones control growth, sexual development, sexual function, reproduction, body temperature, and energy regulation. An error in the production or release of hormones can cause serious health problems.

Hormones are produced and released in daily cycles. Some hormones are released *during certain stages of sleep*. For example, approximately 80 percent of all growth hormone is released shortly after sleep begins and is most prominent during the deepest stages of sleep. In fact, sleep seems to modulate the release of this hormone. If sleep does not occur, neither does growth hormone secretion. If sleep is postponed, the secretion of growth hormone is also postponed, altering its daily, rhythmic cycle. So when your mother told you that you would stunt your growth by staying up late, she spoke with a grain of truth.

Another example of a hormone related to sleep is noradrenaline, which helps regulate wakefulness and alertness. Noradrenaline levels are high during the day and normally are low throughout the sleep period. Sleep deprivation prevents this drop in noradrenaline.

Though research has documented that such hormonal changes exist, we still don't know their impact on our mental and physical condition. Some researchers have hypothesized that a link exists between hormone secretion and the uncomfortable physical symptoms commonly associated with jet lag.

Could the hormonal changes that follow sleep deprivation cause serious problems? It's possible. However, to date we have little scientific evidence to suggest that sleep deprivation causes significant, long-standing hormonal deficiencies.

Sleep and the Immune System

The immune system defends the body against invaders such as viruses, bacteria, and other harmful substances. In the past several years, scientists have been investigating the possibility that sleep deprivation suppresses this complex system.

In one study, researchers looked at whether sleep deprivation reduced the ability of mice to fight off respiratory disease. The researchers found that sleep-deprived, immunized mice were as vulnerable to the flu as if they had never had their shot.

Of course, people are not mice. The idea that sleep deprivation may make humans more vulnerable to viral infections, such as the common cold or flu, is controversial. Some studies have shown an increase in susceptibility to colds following sleep deprivation. However, some scientists think the true culprit is stress that is precipitating both the insomnia and the reduced immunity. Many sleep-deprived people are very active and under stress during periods of sleep loss. Some data suggest that when sleep-deprived people are not under stress, the sleep loss has little influence on the immune system.

The notion that sleep deprivation is related to immune function has led to another question: Could sleep deprivation make someone more susceptible to serious infectious diseases? The evidence is still slight, but some studies indicate that the answer may be yes. A recent study of depressed people showed that sleep deprivation reduced by 28 percent the activity of the body's natural "killer cells," which kill substances that pose a threat to the body. When normal sleep resumed, the natural-killer-cell activity returned to normal. These findings suggest that sleep is vital to regulation of immunity and that even a modest disturbance of sleep reduces it. Other studies of animals and of humans have suggested that a breakdown in defenses against infection follows sleep deprivation.

Accidents

Probably the greatest danger posed by sleep deprivation happens on our highways. Any sleep-deprived person who operates a motor vehicle puts both himself or herself, and other people, at risk.

Andrew Pack believes that he survived such an accident so he could tell others about the dangers of driving when sleepy. In the summer of 1993, everything was going as planned in his life. He was getting ready for his junior year at LaSalle University, was working two jobs, and was occasionally driving to the shore. On August 6, something happened that would change his life and take another. Midafternoon, he fell asleep at the wheel. His car swerved into the next lane and collided head on with an oncoming car, killing the driver instantly. Pack had serious injuries. Today, he dedicates himself to being a public advocate against driving when drowsy.

The time of day that Pack's accident occurred, midafternoon, is one of two times when the body's internal clock makes us sleepy. The other time is the hours after midnight. These are the two most dangerous times to be driving, especially if you haven't had enough sleep. If you have sleep deprivation, you may fall asleep at the wheel no matter how hard you try not to.

Professional drivers who spend long hours on the road are also at risk. Recent research suggests that many long-haul truckers have disturbed sleep and sleep deprivation. In addition to the risk of driving without adequate sleep the night before, many long-haul truckers have some degree of sleep apnea (eight out of ten, according to a study conducted at Stanford University)!

Besides driving, other activities also pose risks both for a sleep-deprived person and others—sometimes many others. Consider the dangers that can be caused by a sleep-deprived pilot, air traffic controller, fire fighter, police officer, doctor, nurse, or child care worker.

Severe sleep deprivation was implicated in the death of Libby Zion, an eighteen-year-old woman who died shortly after being admitted to the New York Hospital–Cornell University Medical Center. In treating Ms. Zion, the staff administered medication that proved lethal in combination with some drugs she had already taken. A grand jury later found that multiple factors were involved, *including the number of hours that interns and residents were required to work.* These work demands can interfere with sleep time. One study conducted in the late 1980s showed that first-year medical residents averaged just 2.6 hours of sleep a day.

Sometimes the consequences of sleep deprivation affect hundreds or thousands of people. For example, when the Exxon *Valdez* ran aground in Prince Edward's Sound in Alaska, an unprecedented oil spill devastated the wildlife and ecology of the bay. Among several probable causes for the grounding of the tanker was crew fatigue. The National Transportation and Safety Board found that no rested deck officer was available to stand watch while the ship sailed through the sound. Sleepiness is also thought to have been one contributor to the accidents involving Three Mile Island, Bhopal, and the space shuttle *Challenger.*

You may have picked up this book because you are just plain frustrated that you're having trouble sleeping or because someone in your life is sleep deprived and the problem is eating away at your relationship. But by solving your sleep problem, you may also make a difference in many other lives. Sleep deprivation is much more than just a personal misery.

ARE YOU AT HIGH RISK FOR SLEEP DEPRIVATION?

Do you think *you* are sleep deprived? Statistically, there's a good chance that you are, because sleep deprivation is an increasingly common experience in our twenty-four-hour-a-day culture.

However, many of the people I see in my practice aren't convinced that they suffer from sleep deprivation. They come to me because their health provider referred them, because their significant other has nagged them into it, or because they know something is wrong and they're checking out all the possibilities, although they're quite certain the problem couldn't be anything as "mundane" as sleep deprivation. Actually, they're expecting to hear a horrible, complicated diagnosis.

Other people I see are convinced that they suffer from sleep deprivation. They know something is lacking in the quantity or quality of their sleep. However, these people often wonder why their nights are so disturbed and their days are so troubled when they allow themselves ample opportunity to sleep at night.

Although some people are referred to me by their doctors, others come to the sleep center on their own after feeling that their doctor has dismissed their sleep problems as unimportant. This situation is not unusual, as most doctors have had little or no training in treating sleep problems. A recent survey of 126 accredited medical schools in the United States revealed that less than two hours of total teaching time is allocated to sleep and sleep disorders during the entire four years of medical school. Thirty-seven schools (29 percent of the sample) reported *no* structured teaching time in this area whatsoever.

Physician education in sleep and sleep disorders is seriously inadequate. Consequently, if you go to your physician with symptoms or complaints related to sleep deprivation, he or she may not know about the high prevalence of this problem, may have no idea of the possible diagnostic strategies, and may not know how to treat the problem appropriately.

When was the last time your health provider asked about your sleep habits? If you bring a problem up, chances are that you will get a quick word of advice or a prescription for a sleep medication. This lack of training makes it all the more important that you take action yourself.

Telling Questions

As the first step on your journey to good nights, ask yourself the following questions to see if you are in a high-risk group for sleep deprivation. Yes or No:

1. Do you need to take a nap during the day?
2. Do you feel sleepy and lack alertness during the day, particularly at boring or monotonous times?
3. Are you a young adult?
4. Are you over 65?
5. Do you have physical, mental, or emotional problems? And do you take medications for these?

Let's look at your answers.
1. Napping can be a sign of sleep deprivation. If you answered yes, you have lots of company. Overall, about 30 percent of people nap frequently—that's almost one in three Americans, more than 160 million people, dozing off during the day.
2. If you answered yes to the second question but don't think you have sleep deprivation, you may be living in denial. Many people attribute daytime sleepiness to other causes, such as a boring lecture, a long stretch of road, or a tedious task. None of these situations causes sleepiness. They only unmask it.
3. If you are a young adult, you're more likely to deny that you have sleep deprivation. Among young adults who don't believe that they

suffer from the effects of sleep deprivation, at least 80 percent show significant daytime symptoms.

4. Older people, while more likely to admit they have trouble sleeping, are also more likely to have sleep deprivation and are more strongly affected by it.

5. In addition to the millions of people who suffer from insufficient sleep for lifestyle reasons, many have insomnia, sleep disorders, medical disorders, psychiatric problems, or other problems that interfere with sleep. If you have physical, mental, or emotional problems, you are at increased risk of sleep deprivation. Many medications can also interfere with sleep.

If you *are* suffering from sleep deprivation, getting the right amount of sound sleep will do more for your health, happiness, and safety than any diet, exercise regime, herb, health food, or vitamin. The good news is that medically proven ways of dealing with your problem are available. You *can* get the sleep that you need, whether the source of your problem is a serious underlying medical condition or simply your attitude toward sleep.

✳ 2 ✳

Sleep Cycles

To understand the nature of normal, restful sleep and what can go wrong, it's very helpful to know about the activity that goes on while we are sleeping. While we think of sleep as rest, for the brain this is a busy, active time. Let's spend a day and night with Sally, a typically harassed and sleep-deprived person who might seem quite familiar to you.

A DAY AND NIGHT WITH SALLY

From the moment Sally was awakened by her alarm, it was another hectic day. A quick cup of coffee, a bowl of cold cereal, then out the door and into the car, driving a little faster than usual because the gas gauge was batting E and she had to stop and fill up on the way to work.

Ten minutes late, she slipped past the boss's door and, to alleviate the nagging guilt for arriving late, worked industriously all morning, skipping the usual midmorning chats at the coffee station.

Just before leaving for lunch, Sally wrote checks for the mortgage and electric and gas bills; then on the way to a sandwich shop, she dropped them in the mailbox in front of the post office. After a long wait to get her lunch at the counter, she ravenously ate her sandwich and then ran over to the nearby bookstore to pick up a recent novel.

She made it back to her desk just in time. For dessert her boss was serving lemon harangue pie. Sally smiled and nodded a lot. After the boss left, Sally shuffled papers, actually managed to solve a problem, and then joined the evening rush, which was no worse than usual. She made the trip pleasant by switching from the nerve-jarring traffic reports to some music that she really enjoyed.

At home she reached into the mailbox and found late notices for the mortgage, electric, and gas bills. She tossed these into the trash basket, did some stretches, and rode on her exercise bike to untie the knots in her neck and shoulders.

On the way to the shower, she raided the refrigerator, finding cold, sliced chicken (How long has it been in here? Smells all right . . .) and an assortment of veggies, which she plunked in the steamer. The steamer shut itself off as she emerged from the shower, wrapped in a cozy old bathrobe.

After supper, Sally put the dishes in the dishwasher, called her mother, puttered around the house a little, ironed slacks for the next day, and then pulled out the novel to read it in bed. By the end of chapter two her eyes were slamming shut, so she got up, checked the doors to be sure they were locked, turned on the dishwasher, turned off the lights, and got back into bed. Listening to the swish of the dishwasher two rooms away, she snuggled into the sheets that smelled of her favorite brand of fabric softener, felt warmth spreading upward from her toes under the comforter, and closed her eyes.

Before the first cycle of the dishwasher had ended, Sally had relaxed completely and hovered in the fog bank that lies between wakefulness and sleep. It felt like her brain was shutting down, shutting, shut . . . but nothing could be farther from the truth, because actually, Sally's brain was just gearing up for a busy night, carrying out some of its most important functions.

Since we just happen to have an electroencephalograph, a machine that measures the electrical activity of the brain and records it on a graph, let's quietly put it on Sally's nightstand, and very carefully, so we don't wake her, attach the electrodes to her head. If we had done this earlier—about half-way through chapter two of her novel—

we would have seen Sally's busy-day brain wave pattern switch to a low-voltage, fast, and rhythmic type of activity, or alpha waves—the kind of waves seen in people who are laying awake motionless with eyes closed, thinking, concentrating, or meditating.

A bit later, Sally is no longer aware of the sound of the dishwasher, so she is entering a transitional state of light sleep, or Stage 1 sleep. It's remarkable how people who enter Stage 1, one of the early stages of sleep, are immediately cut off from the external world. They fail to respond to visual stimuli, and it takes more aggressive sound and sensory stimulation to awaken them. If we had some other instruments available, we'd see that Sally's body is turning down other activities, causing a drop in her heart rate, respiration rate, and blood pressure.

Whoops, there goes the phone. It's her mother. Sally tells her truthfully—but mistakenly—that no, she wasn't asleep when the phone rang. (When people in Stage 1 sleep are awakened and asked to provide a report, many will claim that they were fully awake, perhaps thinking about some important topic.)

"Did you remember to pay the gas and electric bill?"

Sally is glad she hadn't told her the mortgage was late, too. "Yes, Mom, I mailed the checks at lunch time. But thanks for reminding me. Good night, sleep tight."

Sally hangs up the phone and closes her eyes. Although she's feeling guilty over the sarcastic tone she used with her mother, our machine shows that she soon reenters Stage 1, and then Stage 2, sleep, and a different brain wave pattern emerges. But sleep is still not deep. At the sound of a pot suddenly clanging in the dishwasher, Sally remains motionless, but her brain responds to the sound with a unique type of brain activity.

Within the first hour of sleep, Sally's brain activity switches again, this time to high-voltage, low-frequency rhythms, producing delta waves, a sure sign of Stages 3 and 4, the deepest stages of sleep. During these stages, thousands of nerve cells in Sally's brain fire in synchrony, like a huge symphony conducted by a masterful artist. Something in the dishwasher has jammed, and the whole machine is shuddering—but Sally hears nothing. She remains totally focused on that symphony, on the restorative work that is going on in her brain.

About nintey minutes pass, and Sally enters the REM period of sleep (Rapid Eye Movement sleep), in which dreams occur. Although her eyes are closed and her muscles are almost entirely still, Sally's eyes are moving rapidly, indicating that she is dreaming. Thanks to a defense system in Sally's brain, though she dreams that she is waving her arms wildly at her boss, her arms remain perfectly still, but she may be breathing faster and her heart rate may be increasing or decreasing as she and her boss continue to squabble. A drop in muscle activity during REM sleep prevents us from acting out our dreams!

This first period of REM sleep lasts only five or ten minutes and concludes Sally's first sleep cycle of the night. As the night continues, the cycle will be repeated, perhaps five or more times, while Sally sleeps for eight hours. With the waning of the night, however, each successive cycle contains less deep sleep and more REM sleep.

Well, it's time for Sally to get up. Jarred awake by her alarm, she may remember dreaming. Had she been awakened earlier in the sleep period, she might not have been aware of dreaming. Though she awakened with the help of the alarm clock, she's had enough sleep this time and is well prepared for another busy day.

Sally needs to get a good night's sleep like this one more often. Although Sally doesn't know it, she might not have been late with those bills if she had made a habit of sleeping well. In the months prior to this one good night of sleep, Sally had allowed several activities to keep her up at night. As a board member of a local charity, Sally had spent hours and hours at a series of evening meetings. Arriving home late, feeling "wired," she had fallen in the habit of watching the late-night talk shows. On two weekends in a row, relatives had come to visit, and Sally had sat up with them into the wee hours catching up on family news. And just six weeks ago, Sally's beloved cat had died, depriving Sally of treasured companionship and a purring lullaby in her ear each night. Ignoring the pleas from her body for a good night's rest, Sally was coming into work late many mornings, and she wasn't performing up to par (one reason her boss was so touchy). She was forgetting important things, was short with people she loved, and looked like hell.

Like Sally, most of us are so accustomed to living as if sleep were optional or expendable that we have no sense of the terrible chances we are taking. Sally was driving when her brain and body were closer to E than her gas tank was.

Mapping Sleep with an EEG

One tool that has helped sleep scientists learn so much about brain activity at night is the electroencephalogram, or EEG. This machine monitors the combined electrical activity of billions of brain cells in the cerebral cortex, through small sensors called electrodes on the surface of the scalp.

EEGs have not only led to many important insights into the stages of sleep but also are used by sleep specialists to diagnose sleep problems. An evaluation of a sleep problem in a clinic may include an overnight hooked up to an EEG machine.

To perform an EEG (which by the way is painless—no shocks involved), electrodes are placed on the scalp with an adhesive gel and attached by wire to the EEG machine. The EEG machine amplifies the electrical signal and sends information to a moving scroll of graph paper or a computer. The electrical activity shows up as a series of waves of various sizes. By looking at the wavelength (the length of an individual wave from its beginning to its end), wave amplitude (the height and depth of the wave, above and below a midpoint on the graph), wave frequency (how often the waves are repeating), and wave patterns, we can tell a great deal about the depth, or stage, of sleep and any sleep disorders that are present.

The stages of sleep show up on an EEG printout like this:

- Relaxed wakefulness (also meditation)—low-voltage, fast waves
- Stage 1 (transitional sleep)—low-voltage, mixed-frequency waves
- Stage 2—low- or mixed-voltage, mixed-frequency rhythm accompanied by unique waves known as K-complexes and by half-second bursts of very fast activity known as sleep spindles
- Stages 3 and 4 (deep sleep)—high-amplitude, slow delta waves
- REM sleep (dreams)—low-voltage, mixed-frequency pattern

SLEEP ARCHITECTURE

Just as a building is constructed of components that must come together in a certain order, the five stages of sleep occur in a characteristic pattern called "sleep architecture." In most adults:

- The night begins with a brief period of Stage 1 (transitional) sleep.
- This is followed by several minutes of Stage 2 sleep.
- Gradually, and usually within the first hour of sleep, Stages 3 and 4 (delta) sleep occur.
- After about ninety minutes, the first REM appears.

It's amazing to watch the occurrence of REM sleep on an EEG monitor. The rhythm changes from the high-amplitude, slow wave activity of delta sleep to the low-voltage, random activity of REM sleep. Eye movements are often prominent and can be discerned easily on an eye-movement recording. It is quite likely that the sleeper is dreaming.

The first REM period of the night is usually short, perhaps only five or ten minutes. When this episode is over, we know that the sleeper has concluded the first sleep cycle of the night.

As the night continues, the sleeper will have several more sleep cycles. A normal sleeper who sleeps for eight hours or longer is likely to have five or more sleep cycles. As the night wears on, each successive cycle is likely to contain less delta sleep and greater amounts of REM sleep.

By the end of the night, the sleeper is likely to be alternating between Stages 1, 2, and REM. The REM sleep episodes are between twenty and thirty minutes long, which is why most of us are more likely to be aware of dreaming when we awaken in the morning than if we awaken earlier in the sleep period.

The average adult sleeps, on average, seven or eight hours per day, regardless of the social, cultural, or environmental situation. However, the range of normal amounts of sleep is tremendous. Some individuals sleep as little as four hours per night; others sleep ten or more.

When Sleep Is Disrupted

Some people sleep for seven, eight, or even more hours a night, but find that their sleep does not restore them. The reason may be that they are spending too much time in the lighter stages of sleep and not enough in the deep stages and REM periods. This happens when something repeatedly arouses them from sleep—perhaps not enough to bring them to consciousness, but enough to shift them to a lighter stage of sleep. Arousals from sleep can be caused by a sudden, loud noise; snoring; sleep apnea; pain from a medical disorder; or many other factors.

We don't know exactly why spending too much time in lighter stages of sleep makes such a difference, but both sleep specialists and the affected people know that it does. As you'll recall, the brain's nerve cells are busiest during those deeper stages. Whatever it is the nerve cells are doing, it's important, because if a person is deprived of deep sleep, the body tries to catch up the next night by entering deep sleep right away.

Your brain will also be missing out on important restorative work if you don't get enough REM sleep. Arousals or awakenings from REM sleep that result in REM deprivation can also cause a pressure to obtain more REM the next time you sleep.

So the quality of your night's sleep depends not only on its length but also on how much deep and REM sleep it contains.

Does Sleep Architecture Change with Age?

As people grow older, they are much more likely to awaken during the night or to rise very early. Many people mistakenly believe they need less sleep, or are incapable of sleeping as well, as they grow older, but actually the architecture of sleep does not change as much as previously believed. Studies have found that older people may experience a bit more wakefulness during the night and have less deep

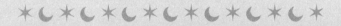

In a Trance

During the transitional stage at the beginning of sleep, it is common to experience visual, dreamlike imagery. At times people experience these hallucinations as though they were fully awake and believe them to be real. If aroused, the individual may be startled to find that the "real" images no longer exist. Some people enjoy this trance-like state and use it as a form of meditation, introspection, or entertainment. Other people experience these hallucinations as dreaming and, if they are aroused, will report that they must have been deeply asleep because they were dreaming.

sleep. But they are entirely capable of having good, healthy sleep. Aging does not necessarily mean that sleep deteriorates.

Studies have also found that sleep deprivation affects older people more than it affects younger people—sleep-deprived older people show greater declines in persistence, attention, precision, and the ability to think and reason. Such effects of sleep deprivation are sometimes misinterpreted as an irreversible mental decline.

Many older people suffer from disrupted sleep not because their biology has changed, but because their health or lifestyle has changed. Among the common culprits are

- Health problems that wake them up such as arthritis, enlarged prostate, and night sweats from menopause
- A greater likelihood of sleep disorders such as sleep apnea and snoring (snoring affects 60 percent of men and 40 percent of women in their sixties)
- Depression or anxiety (each more common at that age)
- Opportunities for daytime napping, which can help fill the sleep need but may also lead to restless sleep or insomnia at night
- Taking more medications for various health problems, increasing the chance that a drug will affect sleep

Whatever the cause or causes of sleep problems, older people can greatly improve their quality of life by getting the sleep they need. Sleep deprivation is not an inevitable part of growing older. It is not your biological destiny.

⋆ 3 ⋆

What's Keeping You Up at Night?

You are now ready to develop some theories about the possible cause or causes of your sleep problem. This prospect may seem intimidating. After all, hundreds of sleep specialists across the country spend their days and nights working with their patients to evaluate and identify the underlying causes of sleep deprivation. However, no amount of study can equip a specialist to know you as well as you know yourself. Armed with the key facts presented here, you can begin to identify your own sleep problems and then take steps to correct them.

If your problem hangs on, even after working through this book or if you feel the input of a specialist would be helpful for any reason, by all means see one promptly. (See chapter 11 for information on how to find a sleep specialist). Also, if it's been more than a year since your last physical, you should have one, including some basic tests, to be sure that no hidden health problems will affect your ability to sleep or to improve your sleep habits.

The sources of sleep problems are divided in this chapter into four groups: insufficient sleep, insomnia, sleep disorders, and medical disorders. Read all four sections, even if your first impression is that they can't possibly apply to you. A questionnaire at the end of this chapter will help you identify, in a general way, the types of sleep problems that you are experiencing and possible contributing factors.

As you enter this process of discovery, keep in mind that there will be few precise or final answers. Your situation may be clear cut or complex. You may suffer from more than one type of disorder or problem that is associated with sleep deprivation. It's more important to establish several good, educated guesses regarding the origin of your sleep problem than to struggle to establish a single cause.

INSUFFICIENT SLEEP

Insufficient sleep is the most common cause of sleep deprivation. Its characteristics are a total daily sleep time that is inadequate to meet sleep needs, excessive daytime sleepiness, and a tendency to sleep longer on weekends or vacations. When a person who's getting insufficient sleep sleeps longer, daytime alertness and functioning improve.

The signs of insufficient sleep are

- You habitually sleep for less time than you think you need.
- You are excessively sleepy during the day.
- You sometimes fall asleep during the day without planning to.
- You sleep longer on weekends or vacations and then awaken spontaneously.
- The symptoms are eliminated by longer sleep periods.
- The troublesome sleep pattern has lasted at least three months.
- No medical, psychiatric, or sleep disorder accounts for the symptoms.

Insufficient sleep is simply a pattern of getting less sleep than is needed to stay alert during the day. It may have happened deliberately (you purposely devote your sleep time to other activities), or it may sneak up on you. People who sleep insufficiently can be aware that they aren't getting the sleep they need, but are often not aware that they subtly and chronically deprive themselves of small amounts of sleep over long periods of time. As the sleep debt mounts, the debilitating effects of sleep loss gradually increase. The person experiences fatigue, sleepiness, mood changes, and functional impairment but, because the process is so slow and gradual, fails to blame sleep deprivation. Many people try diets, exercise, nutritional supplements, rest (but not sleep), or other remedies with absolutely no improvement because they're not addressing the real problem.

Two Tales of Insufficient Sleep

Donna's wake-up call came in a very troubling way. A thirty-year-old married mother of three, she worked full-time as a surgical assistant in one of her town's busiest hospitals. In recent months, Donna had become increasingly aware she wasn't able to perform her usual activities at home—and then she made a serious error in the operating room, one that could have injured a patient.

Several days later, Donna saw her physician, who sent her to us at the sleep center. Both Donna's husband and her employer asked her to take time off from work to get the evaluation done.

When I interviewed Donna, there was no question that she was suffering from insufficient sleep. Her day typically started early, before six A.M., when she rose to prepare for work and get her children ready for school. Once at work, Donna immediately prepared the operating room for the first surgical case of the morning and then remained present for the operation. She attended to her professional tasks with great care and devotion and had earned the reputation of being one of the best surgical assistants at the hospital.

After this exhausting round of activities, Donna drove home just in time to meet her children as they came home from school and began her "second shift" of cleaning, laundry, shopping, and the million little details that go into raising children well. Donna was an excellent cook and was proud of the delicious meals that she prepared each night for her family.

After dinner, it was time to clean the kitchen, monitor the children's homework, get them into bed, and finally, take care of any remaining business of the day. Her last task of the night, often well after midnight, was to lay out the children's clothing for the next day. Her own bedtime was routinely delayed until one A.M. As is typical in our culture, people responded to Donna's endless days and inadequate sleep with admiration, frequently commenting on her capabilities as a wife, mother, homemaker, and professional. Her family and friends called her "Wonder Woman."

When she first became aware of feeling tired, it didn't occur to Donna that her sleep patterns could be the source. She thought she was nipping just a little off her sleep schedule, to fit a day-and-a-half of work into each day, but actually she had had only five hours of sleep a night for several months. Night after night, she had deprived herself of the sleep she needed. Her fatigue, errors on the job, and darkening mood were signs that her schedule had caught up with her.

Robert's story is another example of insufficient sleep. When I first met him, Robert was a forty-three-year-old, divorced building contractor who was supervising the construction of a large office and apartment tower in mid-Manhattan. He complained of feeling sleepy and unable to perform at peak during the day, noting that Thursdays and Fridays were absolutely his worst days: "I end the week feeling exhausted." Recently, Robert had been forced to take occasional afternoon naps before he could complete his paperwork at the end of the day without making many errors or falling asleep at his desk. He was aware of becoming irritable and abrasive with his coworkers and of using poor judgment at times. Unable to identify the cause of his problems, he visited his doctor.

Robert normally rose each day at five A.M. He felt sleepy on awakening but tended to feel better after he showered and dressed. A coffee lover, Robert would stop at a coffee shop on the way to work, filling his thermos with a special blend. He frankly admitted that caffeine gave him the extra boost that he needed to get through the morning.

Like Donna, Robert loved his job. He arrived at the construction site by 6:30 and worked hard all day. He often remained to tie up loose ends long after the work crew had gone home. Afterward, he might visit with his children, a boy of five and a girl of seven, or he might go out for dinner with male friends or his girlfriend. Upon returning home, Robert typically retired at eleven P.M., fell asleep quickly, and remained asleep until his morning alarm. His difficulty arising in the morning worsened as the work week wore on, but on the weekends he allowed himself to sleep until about ten or eleven A.M. and had no trouble getting up.

Clearly, Robert was chronically and unknowingly sleep deprived and suffered from insufficient sleep. Although he slept solidly for six hours per night, I was certain that this amount of sleep was not adequate for him because on most mornings he awoke feeling tired, he required coffee to raise his level of alertness and performance, and he felt fatigued and sleepy later in the day. His weekend sleep-ins accounted for about five hours more sleep than he would get on a work day, an obvious attempt to recover lost sleep. Since Robert was refreshed following long sleep bouts on the weekend, he started the week feeling better but was dragging again by the end of the week. Yet Robert had no clue that his total nightly sleep time during the week was inadequate.

If You Suspect Your Problem Is Insufficient Sleep

Insufficient sleep often develops so slowly and subtly that just recognizing that you have this problem is an important step toward finding solutions. Remember: *The primary and most profound effect of insufficient sleep is excessive or nagging daytime sleepiness. An adequate amount of sleep will enable the sleeper to feel alert during normal hours of wakefulness. In the absence of a medical, psychiatric, or sleep disorder, sleepiness during normal hours of wakefulness, persisting for three months or more, is probably caused by insufficient sleep.*

The solution to insufficient sleep is, of course, getting sufficient sleep! The key is to find out how much sleep you need, and then to establish a schedule that will help you get that number of hours, night after night. Chapter 4 will tell you how.

INSOMNIA

Another cause of sleep deprivation is insomnia, a sleep disorder defined as difficulty falling asleep, difficulty staying asleep, or early morning awakening. Insomnia not only is the most common sleep disorder but also is one of the most prevalent health disorders of any kind in our society. A 1995 Gallup telephone survey of 1,027 adult men and women eighteen and over revealed that about 49 percent of the adult population of the United States suffers from at least occasional insomnia; 12 percent reported that their insomnia is chronic and frequent. More than seventy million Americans have experienced occasional insomnia, and for twenty million, the problem is chronic. A staggering amount of tossing and turning is going on in our bedrooms each night.

The most common type of insomnia, *transient insomnia*, lasts one or two nights and is usually a response to a particular emotional, mental, or physical stress. *Any* stressful life event, even a minor one, can provoke insomnia: a disagreement with a spouse, a bad day at work, financial concerns, or a physical ailment or injury, to name a few. A joyful event—a pending wedding, for example, or an anticipated visit from a long-absent loved one—may trigger sleeplessness that can leave you just as fatigued as insomnia caused by unfortunate events.

Short-term insomnia lasts from several days to several weeks and usually is caused by some temporary misery, perhaps a disagreement with a boss or a brief illness. Short-term insomnia often improves or goes away when the cause of the stress is resolved or ends.

Eric, an accountant, developed a classic case of short-term insomnia when he was preparing for an audit of his company's records. The pressure to work accurately and quickly was overwhelming, and the hours were long and deadly tedious. The first signs of trouble were a sour stomach from fast-food dinners and irritability caused by separation from his family and normal routine. Not surprisingly, Eric developed terrible short-term insomnia that kept him up night after night. Of course, not being able to restore himself through sleep made his job situation worse. Frustrating errors cropped up, even in simple addition and subtraction calculations. Tired and anxious, Eric felt as if he were trapped in insomnia for life, but a few days after the audit was over, his sleep was almost back to normal.

If you suffer from transient or short-term insomnia, your symptoms may improve if you deal with any underlying stress. For example, if insomnia is the result of stress at work, reducing that stress often resolves the insomnia. Besides stress, other possible precipitating factors are a change in the environment, medical problems, psychiatric problems, alcohol or drug problems, and some prescription medications (including appropriately prescribed medicines taken exactly as the physician recommended).

If stress has prompted some nights or weeks of insomnia, it is important that you guard against the insidious development of a long-term problem. Insomnia that lasts from several weeks to several years is called *chronic insomnia*. For most people with chronic insomnia, a visit with the doctor to discuss insomnia comes only after many years of misery. In the Gallup survey mentioned above, the average duration of the sleep problem was eleven years! Although chronic insomnia often begins at a stressful time, it can begin without an obvious cause. In either case, chronic insomnia takes on a life of its own. You can tell that you are on the way to chronic insomnia if you deal effectively with the source of the stress or other problem and the insomnia still hangs on. In this situation, it's unrealistic to expect that your symptoms will eventually just simply go away. You will have to take action to remedy the problem.

Regardless of whether it is transient, short-term, or chronic, insomnia includes one or more of the following:

- **Difficulty falling asleep.** You lie awake thirty minutes or longer after turning out the lights.
- **Difficulty staying asleep.** You wake up many times, or for a long time, during the sleep period. You may awaken as many as twenty times per night and find it difficult to return to sleep. Even one awakening can cause sleep deprivation if you stay awake long enough.
- **Early morning awakenings.** You wake up near the end of the sleep period but earlier than you want to—perhaps at four or five A.M.—and then find it difficult or impossible to return to sleep.

Most people with chronic insomnia report more than one of the preceding symptoms. About 49 percent report difficulty falling asleep, 68 percent report many awakenings during the night, and 25 percent report difficulty returning to sleep if they should awaken during the night or wake up too early. If you add up the percentages, the total is more than 100 percent, showing that most people with insomnia have trouble both falling asleep and staying asleep.

Unfortunately, each time you get into bed and have difficulty falling asleep, or wake up and lie awake in bed, you are strengthening the association between wakefulness and your sleep environment. People should feel relaxed and comfortable while lying in bed awaiting sleep. If insomnia continues, soon you will associate your sleep environment with wakefulness, agitation, frustration, and other reactions that are incompatible with sleep. Instead of becoming increasingly ready for sleep, you may become hyperaroused and ready for another fitful night.

Insomnia often prompts feelings and thoughts that make it difficult to fall asleep:

- **Fear.** If you have insomnia, you may dread the coming night. Some people with insomnia spend the hours before bedtime gripped with a silent but mounting fear of experiencing the insomnia on yet another night. They feel helpless to overcome their fear.

- **Worry.** You may worry about how you will function the next day.
- **Frustration.** You may become frustrated that you cannot control your sleep.
- **Disturbing thoughts.** Periods of wakefulness during the night may swell with the weighty concerns of the day. You may begin to think about troubles at home or at work, things that were done or not done during the day, financial problems, health concerns, or any number of disruptive thoughts. Your thinking is usually not productive. (I remember one sleepless night of my own during which I lamented a comment that I had made to a colleague regarding his work. I was certain that he had misinterpreted my comment as an insult. When I approached him about it the next day, I learned that he had not even heard what I had said, let alone been affronted by it.)
- **Depression and anxiety.** Periods of wakefulness during the night can become associated with a low mood or anxiety. For some people, the depression becomes so severe that situations in their lives seem hopeless. People who have anxiety disorders can suffer panic attacks as they lie awake in bed.
- **Behavior incompatible with sleep.** It may be tempting to occupy your wakeful nights with activity: watching television or listening to the radio in bed, reading, talking on the telephone (thus sharing your sleeplessness with a friend!), eating, paying bills, cleaning house, walking the dog, taking out the garbage. But stimulating activities of any kind, even quiet ones, may make it harder for you to return to sleep when you return to bed.

So insomnia is not just sleeplessness. It's sleeplessness plus a complex combination of fear, worry, frustration, disturbing thoughts, mood changes, and disruptive behaviors—and these are just the *nighttime* symptoms.

During the day, people suffer from both fatigue and sleepiness. Fatigue is a physical, emotional, or mental state of being "run down" or exhausted. Sleepiness refers to the drive to sleep—to feel drowsy, to doze off, or to nap.

Some people with insomnia get up feeling washed out and exhausted and ramble through the entire day in this condition. Just as they can't sleep at night, they can't sleep during the day, so they can't use naps to help them feel better. For these people, life becomes an endless cycle of bad nights and long, miserable days. Other people with insomnia may be sleepy. They may nod off at meetings, while listening to the boss drone on about something, or at other inappropriate times.

Whether from fatigue, sleepiness, or both, people with insomnia often suffer from impaired performance during the day. The result can be small nuisances, such as misplacing an object or incorrectly dialing a telephone number, or a significant problem, such as erasing forever a vital computer file. There can be more memory problems, more difficulty coping with day-to-day stresses, and more difficulty completing simple tasks. These effects can markedly affect one's ability to function at home and work. For example, a University of Michigan survey of 1,445 employees found that insomnia was a better predictor of absenteeism than were obesity, job-caused injury, disability, or back pain! People with chronic insomnia are 2.5 times more likely to be involved in a fatigue-related automobile accident than are people with no insomnia. If the person works as an air-traffic controller, a pilot, a bus driver, a surgeon, or an operator at a power plant, even minor impairments in performance can have far-reaching consequences.

A Story of Insomnia

Louise was a middle-aged attorney who had slept well for most of her life. While in her early thirties, she was employed by a firm that specialized in corporate law. Louise was considered an "up and comer" and worked with many of the firm's most important clients.

One client owned a manufacturing company that supplied mate-

* (* (* (* (* (* (* (*

High-Altitude Insomnia

People who travel to places with high altitudes sometimes experience difficulty falling asleep or staying asleep. This problem appears to be related to changes in breathing that occur at altitudes above thirteen thousand feet.

rial for aircraft engines. Louise had established a strong professional relationship with the man, coming to know him and his family on a first-name basis. One year the client was sued after allegedly supplying defective parts to a buyer. This suit threatened to cost his company millions of dollars. This was Louise's first important case representing this client, and it had the potential to advance her position within the firm. The pressure mounted as the case approached trial, and Louise soon found herself overly involved. She frequently worried about her client and his family and how the outcome of the case would affect them.

At about that time, Louise began to experience difficulty falling asleep. She spent several nights awake in bed, wrestling with worry about her professional competence and fears that she would fail. As the court case moved on, her sleep problems worsened. She took longer to fall asleep and could barely get up and get going in the morning. She felt forced to schedule only afternoon and evening appointments with clients. Over several months, the problem lingered.

Louise won the case, but to her frustration the sleep problems hung on. Each night, she lay awake and rehashed the day's events. The longer she stayed in bed, the larger her problems seemed and the angrier she became. Eventually she went to her living room and stretched out on the sofa to watch television, where she would fall asleep between two and three A.M. She would awaken at nine or ten A.M. feeling exhausted. She tried alcohol as a sedative and experimented with home remedies, but these didn't help either.

Louise's diagnosis? Chronic sleep-onset insomnia. Though the stress that started her insomnia had been resolved, her problem persisted. In addition to sleeplessness, Louise experienced frustration and anger, and she engaged in at least one behavior that was incompatible with sleep (lying on the sofa to watch television). The use of alcohol as a sedative probably worsened, rather than improved, her sleep. As you can imagine, insomnia was having an impact on the most vital areas of Louise's life, affecting not only her performance but also her confidence and self-image.

If You Suspect Your Problem Is Insomnia

If your insomnia has lasted only a few days or weeks, you can often resolve it by dealing with the precipitating stress or other problem in your life or by using medication on an as-needed basis. If the insomnia has become chronic, your first step should be to follow the steps in chapter 4 to establish a sleep schedule.

The "ten tips" in chapter 5 will also help to improve your sleep habits. These tips will help you get ready for your night of sleep and will help you change daytime habits that may be affecting your sleep more than you realize. Two tips that particularly warrant your attention concern alcohol and smoking. Many people with chronic insomnia self-medicate with alcohol. Alcohol is a powerful sedative and it may

✳ ☾ ✳ ☾ ✳ ☾ ✳ ☾ ✳ ☾ ✳ ☾ ✳ ☾ ✳

Your Plan for Stopping Insomnia

In the chapters to come, you will learn many techniques for ending insomnia. For best results, apply them in the following order. Of course, if the early steps do the trick, you need not go further. Here's your plan for success:

1. *Read this chapter to check for signs that a sleep disorder or medical problem may be the source of your insomnia. If you suspect an underlying cause, see your doctor or a sleep specialist. Also, if you have not had a medical checkup in over a year, schedule one now.*
2. *Use a sleep log and the sleepiness scale to determine how many hours of sleep you need each night (see chapter 4).*
3. *Set your rise time and bedtime to insure you get adequate sleep and stick with it every day of the week (chapter 4).*
4. *Apply the ten tips for a good night (chapter 5). Make no more than three changes in your sleep habits at a time and stick with each change for at least three weeks before deciding it doesn't work.*
5. *While you are implementing the above changes, talk to your doctor about whether short-term treatment with a sleep medication might support your efforts.*
6. *If necessary, apply a behavioral technique from chapter 6: stimulus control therapy, sleep restriction therapy, a relaxation therapy, or cognitive retraining. Again, a sleeping pill may be part of your overall efforts.*
7. *If you have applied the techniques carefully and faithfully, there's a very good chance your insomnia will be much improved. If you are not getting the results you want, consider treatment at a sleep-disorders center.*

seem to be helping at first. But using alcohol this way can lead to both sleep problems and bigger problems. Drinking in the evening causes lighter, disturbed sleep in the second half of the night. Even more dangerously, this practice can lead to alcohol dependence. In one study, people who had been diagnosed with insomnia were asked three years later whether they used alcohol for sleep. At this time, 3.6 percent said yes. But two years after that, 12.5 percent were using alcohol as a sedative. This is a dangerous pattern!

The other tip I want to bring up here concerns smoking. While most of us know that caffeine is a stimulant and therefore avoid coffee in the evenings, many people don't realize that their cigarettes are equally, if not more, stimulating. If you are a smoker and you are fighting insomnia, getting rid of the cigarette habit would be a good start to better sleep and a longer, healthier life.

If insomnia persists after applying the ten tips and a good sleep schedule, your solution may be a behavioral technique such as relaxation therapy; details appear in chapter 6. When used as part of an overall sleep program, sleep medications can also help break the chain of chronic insomnia. Chapter 7 explains how drugs can be used wisely. Both behavioral techniques and medications work better in the context of a regular sleep period and good sleep habits, so I advise that you use them after you have established a regular bed time and rise time and in conjunction with the ten tips for better sleep.

SLEEP DISORDERS

More than eighty different disorders can disrupt sleep and cause sleep deprivation. Some sleep disorders change the architecture of sleep we talked about in chapter 2 by fragmenting sleep, increasing the amounts of wakefulness and light sleep, or decreasing the amount of deep sleep and REM periods. To help you recognize if your problem is a sleep disorder, read these descriptions and symptoms of the most common problems. You can find more about these and other sleep disorders in chapter 10.

Sleep Apnea

Sleep apnea causes periodic reductions or complete interruptions in airflow during sleep. That's right—the sleeper's breathing stops altogether! Whenever I've observed this phenomenon, moments of silence seem to tick on forever until the brain gets the message that the body's oxygen level is dropping and the sleeper arouses, snorting and snarling for air. Typically, restored by breathing, the resurrected sleeper will drift right back to sleep with no recollection of the events, even when they occur repeatedly during the night.

Apnea events can markedly alter sleep architecture. A person with sleep apnea gets lots of Stage 1 (light) sleep at the expense of the deeper, restorative stages of sleep (Stages 3 and 4 and REM sleep). These folks feel they sleep very poorly—which they do—and many experience the daytime effects of sleep deprivation.

Restless Legs Syndrome

Restless legs syndrome causes unpleasant or painful sensations like tickling, deep aching, or mild to severe muscle spasm in the lower limbs. The feelings occur most often when a person is lying awake in bed right before sleep but can also occur during the night. The person has a strong, almost irresistible impulse to try to relieve the sensations by stretching, flexing, or repositioning the leg, or even walking.

Restless legs syndrome can significantly prolong the start of sleep, as well as the duration of any awakenings during the night. The sleeper remains fully awake or drifts in and out of light sleep.

Periodic Limb Movement Disorder

This puzzling, uncomfortable disorder is characterized by repetitive limb movements, twitches, or jerks that take place during sleep. Some sleepers may experience one or more movements each minute. An EEG shows that the movements are causing arousal in the brain. The disorder increases the amount of light sleep and reduces the deeper stages.

Circadian Rhythm Disorders

These sleep schedule disorders cause periods of sleep to occur at undesirable times. Many people with circadian rhythm disorders obtain adequate amounts of sleep, but because the timing is off, they are awake or sleepy at inappropriate times.

Parasomnias

Parasomnias (the term means "around or about sleep") are abnormal behaviors during sleep, such as sleepwalking, night terrors, nightmares, confusional arousals, enuresis (bedwetting), and REM behavior disorder. These behaviors can lead to sleep deprivation by disrupting sleep or causing awakenings.

If You Suspect Your Problem Is a Sleep Disorder

If you recognize your problem in any of these descriptions, read more about the sleep disorder in chapter 10 and then seek help from your doctor or a sleep specialist. Specific treatments are available, including medications and special devices and therapies. Don't try to solve these problems on your own.

MEDICAL DISORDERS

A wide variety of medical disorders and conditions can lead to sleep deprivation. Chronic pain, heart disease, depression, and many other problems can increase not only the amount of time it takes to fall asleep but also the number of awakenings. The result is an increase in light sleep and reduction in deeper and REM sleep.

If you have pain or physical limitations, your sleep may be disrupted simply because you are unable to get enough exercise, must sit idle for long periods, or must spend excessive time in bed. In this situation, the distinction between appropriate periods of wakefulness and sleep is blurred. Poor sleep habits may develop, leading to insomnia and sleep-schedule problems. Furthermore, when you experience any serious medical problem, worries about your health can invade your nights and result in insomnia.

Coming Home from the Hospital with Insomnia

If your medical condition leads to hospitalization, you suddenly face many new stresses: invasive medical diagnostic or treatment procedures, constant bed rest or limited movement, hospital food on a hospital schedule, a restricted diet, interruptions of sleep for medication, medications that sedate you or make you "hyper," the noise of a hospital environment, and probably the most troublesome of all, separation from your family and daily routine. All these stressful situations can suddenly bring on sleep difficulties and significant sleep deprivation. Surgery itself disrupts sleep very much, even if the pain afterwards is well managed and the environment is kept peaceful. Studies have shown that on average patients spend more than 40 percent of the night following an operation awake or in light sleep. The amount of deeper stages and REM sleep can be negligible.

Mr. Gordon was a classic case of insomnia following hospitalization and surgery. Although he had slept easily all his life, at age seventy-two he developed severe insomnia. When the insomnia continued for four months, he was referred to our sleep-disorders center. He reported that his health had been failing since retirement from his small jeweler's shop and that he had recently undergone heart bypass surgery. Although this surgery is very common today and has a high success rate, it is about as major and intimidating as surgery can get. So, although his heart doctor declared the surgery a great success, Mr. Gordon harbored some doubts. When I met him at the sleep center, he spoke openly about his fear of dying and leaving his wife of forty-two years alone in the world.

Mr. Gordon recalled that the severe insomnia started on the night following the surgery. On that night, he was in some discomfort, despite pain medication, and was unable to move freely. After he lay awake in bed, tossing and turning as much as his condition would allow, one of the nurses brought him a sleep medication. The medication helped, so it was continued during the rest of his hospital stay and when he was sent home. At home the medication was modestly successful at first, but within the first week or two, its effects diminished markedly, so Mr. Gordon stopped using it. Instead, he resorted to lying awake in bed or getting up to drink herbal tea throughout the night. Ultimately, it was taking him more than three hours to fall asleep, he could only sleep for two or three hours before awakening, and he then was unable to return to sleep. He lay awake worrying about his health and his family.

As frequently happens, hospitalization was the start of Mr. Gordon's insomnia. Since the sleep medication helped only for a short time and had been prescribed on an "as needed" basis, he was right to discontinue it when he did; however, he complicated the situation by starting a nighttime ritual, tea drinking, that became a sleep disrupter.

Pain

Pain is a common cause of sleep deprivation. *Acute pain* due to injury or illness can increase the amount of time spent awake in bed during the sleep period. Depending on the severity, pain can also result in disturbed and restless sleep. If you are experiencing pain, you may have increased amounts of light sleep and may even awaken frequently to relieve discomfort by changing position in bed or trying other remedies.

Pain that continues for weeks, months, or years is called *chronic pain.* Chronic pain also disrupts nighttime sleep, sometimes severely. People with chronic pain suffer from long periods of wakefulness before onset of sleep and from increased wakefulness during the night. They can also experience *alpha intrusions,* short bursts of alpha activity in the brain, lasting only a few seconds, that seem to fragment sleep and disrupt sleep architecture. These problems can significantly reduce total sleep time and result in short-term or chronic sleep deprivation.

Arthritis

Arthritis is inflammation of the joints, usually associated with pain ranging from a vague, nagging discomfort to grating, relentless suffering. *Osteoarthritis* is the "wear and tear" arthritis that most people experience in their joints to some degree as they grow older. *Rheumatoid arthritis* is an autoimmune disease that affects the entire body, causing joint inflammation and pain accompanied by symptoms such as fatigue, loss of strength, stiffness, and sometimes fever. Rheumatoid arthritis often leads to crippling deformities.

In both forms of arthritis, the pain is often worse at night, which can increase the time awake in bed and the amount of light sleep. For people with rheumatoid arthritis, this sleeplessness can be doubly detrimental because a vital component of managing the illness is rest and restorative sleep.

Chronic Fatigue Syndrome

Chronic fatigue syndrome is a collection of symptoms that usually includes extreme fatigue and weakness after exertion, flulike symptoms, muscle aches, joint pain, and headache. It is usually diagnosed by ruling out other disorders. The symptoms must have persisted for at least twelve weeks. Often symptoms last for months and are some-times permanent.

Pain and discomfort during the sleep period are common, as are a long period before sleep onset, increased amounts of wakefulness during the sleep period, arousals, alpha intrusions in sleep, and increased amounts of light sleep. (For a definition of alpha intrusions, see the preceding section on pain.) Many people with chronic fatigue syndrome alter the day and night patterns of sleep and wakefulness. When they are experiencing symptoms, they rest or sleep for long periods during the day, inadvertently reducing the likelihood of sleep throughout the night.

Headaches

Headaches are one of the most common of all ailments. Some are associated with a variety of medical illnesses, and others hit people who are fit and healthy.

Tension headaches are mild to substantial miseries that result from stress, such as unexpectedly finding a letter in the mailbox with the return address of a law firm or worrying because a work project is overdue. These headaches normally respond to a pain medication, a short rest or a few minutes of quiet, or opening the letter from the law firm and finding that a little old man you helped across the street has remembered you—substantially—in his will.

Sinus headaches usually begin in the front part of the head or in the face and can escalate to become incredibly painful. They tend to be worse in the morning and in cold, damp weather. Indicators that the headache stems from the sinuses are a recent cold or other upper-respiratory infection, pain in one part of the face, and a greenish nasal discharge.

Migraine headaches are severe and require prompt medical evaluation, isolation (bed rest in a quiet, darkened room), and perhaps prescription medications that are much stronger than over-the-counter pain killers. A classic migraine headache often begins in and around the eyes and includes not only severe, sometimes throbbing pain but also sensitivity to light and sound, loss of appetite, and nausea or vomiting. Migraine headaches frequently become prolonged if they are not treated.

Like migraines, *cluster headaches* are severe and disabling, sometimes for days, but they affect only one side of the temple, neck, or face. Cluster headaches may cause swelling below the affected eye, runny nose, and tearing. Like migraines, cluster headaches tend to be chronic and require careful medical evaluation and treatment.

Migraine and cluster headaches can begin during sleep, usually during the REM period. Sleep-associated headaches can result in insomnia, especially during the early-morning hours when REM sleep is abundant.

Headaches can also be caused by allergies, brain tumors, and other health problems. The sleep disorder called sleep apnea can also cause headaches.

Most people with headaches go a long time between episodes. With good medical management, even migraine and cluster headaches do not happen every day or night. Therefore, headaches are not likely to be the underlying cause of nightly sleep deprivation. However, they can give rise to insomnia. Headaches can prolong the period before sleep onset and can also contribute to awakenings and wakefulness during the sleep period. If headache episodes occur one after the other, they can lead to a significant period of sleep deprivation.

Frequent Urination

Any condition that sends you to the bathroom several times a night will disrupt your sleep. Urinary tract infections are a common problem for women of all ages, and the risk more than triples over age sixty. Also more common among older women is urinary incontinence, which can take the form of leaking or of uncontrollable, sudden urges to void. Among men, the most common cause of frequent urination is an enlarged prostate gland (benign prostatic hypertrophy or BPH), which affects about 75 percent of men over age fifty.

When urinary frequency occurs, the sleeper usually awakens, stumbles to the bathroom, empties the bladder (or tries to—the urge does not always mean that the bladder is full), and returns to bed. For most people, the return to sleep is rapid; however, for those with difficulty falling asleep, several such awakenings during the night can result in long hours of wakefulness during the sleep period. Even if you fall back to sleep right away, awakenings during the night somewhat affect your sleep architecture, though not significantly.

Breathing Disorders

Asthma is a potentially deadly response to a substance to which you are allergic. While we tend to think of asthma as a children's disease, many adults have asthma, and an adult with no history of allergies can suddenly develop it. In a person with asthma, dust, pollen, or some other offending substance triggers attacks in which the bronchial passages that carry air deep into the lungs constrict, cutting off the oxygen supply. As the person struggles to force air through the narrowed passages, there is a characteristic high-pitched whistle called a wheeze. The condition is treated with bronchodilator drugs.

The lungs of a person with *emphysema* become increasingly less efficient because of progressive damage to the air sacs. The main symptom is shortness of breath. The condition is often treated with supplemental oxygen administration.

Both EEG tests and personal reports from sufferers show that breathing disorders like asthma and emphysema fragment sleep, increase wakefulness during the sleep period, and lighten sleep. The sleeper responds to impaired breathing by arousing or awakening. Coughing or wheezing can also wake up the sleeper. Other awakenings are responses to low levels of oxygen or high levels of carbon dioxide.

Heart Disease

Angina is severe, suffocating pain in the chest caused when the oxygen supply to the heart muscle is interrupted. The pain often radiates to the left arm or other parts of the body. Normally, angina occurs during exercise, exertion, or excitement. When it occurs during sleep, the pain may awaken the sleeper. Angina is a warning sign of a potential heart attack, so it should always be reported promptly to your doctor.

Cardiac arrhythmias such as palpitations (rapid, fluttering heartbeats) can also contribute to nighttime awakenings.

Congestive heart failure occurs when the heart pumps inefficiently and may not pump enough blood to the lungs and the rest of the body. Disturbed sleep is common among people with this problem because of an accompanying breathing problem called Cheyne-Stokes respiration. Instead of breathing steadily, with a fairly constant rhythm and volume of air intake and exhalation, a person with Cheyne-Stokes respiration breathes in a pattern that might be pictured as a pyramid. Near the broad base, the cycle begins with a normal breath, but each subsequent breath becomes smaller and shallower, and the amount of oxygen available to the body gets smaller and smaller. Then, suddenly, to compensate, a very large breath must be taken, and the cycle begins again. As you can imagine, this type of breathing leads to frequent arousals and poor sleep.

Coronary artery bypass surgery is infamous for causing sleep problems including severe insomnia. Sleep problems usually peak three to six weeks after surgery.

Gastric (Stomach) Problems

Any kind of gastrointestinal disorder can give rise to sleep disturbances, including a long period before sleep onset, fragmented sleep, frequent arousals or awakenings, or all of the above.

In *peptic ulcer disease*, lesions develop in the stomach. A stomach ache that interferes with sleep is a warning sign of an ulcer. The dull pain usually occurs one to four hours after falling asleep. The pain may radiate into the chest or back and be accompanied by a burning sensation in the stomach or chest and a feeling of fullness, nausea, or cramping. Many arousals from sleep may occur, as well as prolonged wakefulness accompanied by discomfort.

Gastroesophageal reflux is a common problem in which stomach fluid or contents from the stomach are regurgitated into the esophagus or the throat during sleep. In most cases, reflux doesn't lead to full awakening, but some sleepers wake up coughing or choking, with a sour taste in the mouth, nasty burning in the back of the throat, and pain or discomfort in the abdomen or chest. Awakenings may be long and fitful.

Allergies and Toxic Substances

Allergies to substances like ragweed, pollen, dust mites, animal dander, or even certain foods can cause sneezing, tearing, itching, or a runny nose, all symptoms that can disrupt sleep.

Exposure to *toxic substances* such as heavy metals, poisons, or chemicals can be the underlying cause of sleep disruption. One of the most prominent symptoms of lead poisoning (and several other toxins) is stomach pain, which many people dismiss, even as it keeps them

awake, until it becomes serious. While exposure to many of these
toxins is primarily an occupational risk, there are other ways to be exposed—for example, old pipes can leach lead into your drinking
water.

Nervous-System Disorders

Many nerve disorders, including epilepsy, Parkinson's disease, mus-
cular dystrophy, Tourette's syndrome, Huntington's chorea, torsion
dystonia, and Morvan's chorea, increase the number of awakenings,
shifts between the stages of sleep, and the length of Stage 1 sleep and
diminish delta and REM sleep. A person with epilepsy may have seizures
during sleep. Tourette's syndrome increases the likelihood of sleepwalking.

Menstruation, Pregnancy, and Menopause

Menstruation, pregnancy, and menopause aren't disorders, of course,
but they're included here as physical conditions that can affect a woman's
sleep.

Changing hormone levels during the week prior to menstruation
can increase the time it takes to go to sleep or can cause multiple awakenings.

If you become pregnant, expect to crave a lot more sleep than usual
during the first three months. An increased need for sleep begins at
the very start of pregnancy and, in fact, is one of the first signs of
pregnancy. In the last three months as it becomes more difficult to
get comfortable in bed, you may have more trouble going to sleep
and may awaken during the night. There may also be a decrease in
the deepest sleep levels. You may need to get up to go to the bathroom during the night. The baby's movements, your increased weight,
sudden leg cramps, and general discomforts may also disturb your sleep.

During menopause, about three-quarters of women experience hot
flashes, which are sudden, intense increases in body temperature lasting
one to three minutes. Perspiration and heart beat may increase. Hot
flashes that occur during the night, called night sweats, can lead to insomnia and sleep deprivation. Sleep problems can lead in turn to mood
swings and depression. If you are troubled by hot flashes and night
sweats, you may want to talk to your doctor about estrogen replacement therapy, which usually stops the problem in two to four weeks.

Depression

Depression is an overwhelming, utter sadness and despair. Depression guts our interest or pleasure in food, work, leisure activities, sex, and the companionship of people we love. It can cause weight loss, feelings of worthlessness, excessive guilt, and diminished ability to think or concentrate. It perpetuates itself by fostering indecisiveness and rendering us nearly incapable of asking for help. In severe cases, thoughts of death or suicide may occur.

Such signs of depression may go away by themselves after a few days or weeks or can last for months or even years if untreated. Depression triggered by an event such as job loss, divorce, or loss of spouse usually lessens with the passage of time and the support of family, friends, or psychotherapy. Depression that occurs every day for at least two weeks, may or may not have a known cause, and interferes with normal daily activities is called a *major depressive disorder,* and it may need to be treated with a combination of medication and psychotherapy.

Not surprisingly, depression often causes sleep problems. According to the *Diagnostic and Statistical Manual of Mental Disorders,* 40 percent to 60 percent of outpatients with major depression, and up to 90 per-

❈☾✳☾✳☾✳☾✳☾✳☾✳☾✳

Symptoms and Signs of Major Depression

Major depression includes low mood or loss of interest and pleasure for at least two weeks, accompanied by at least four of the following symptoms:

- *Feeling agitated or feeling slowed down*
- *Difficulty concentrating*
- *Sleeplessness or extreme sleepiness*
- *Lack of energy or fatigue*
- *Loss of appetite, weight loss, or weight gain*
- *Guilt and feelings of worthlessness*
- *Thoughts of death or recurrent suicidal ideas*

cent of hospitalized patients, show signs of sleep problems, including an increased length of time before the start of sleep; fragmented sleep, with multiple or long awakenings; early-morning awakenings, usually between four and five A.M.; and reductions in deep and REM sleep.

Not only does depression cause sleep disorders, but sleep problems can make depression worse. Insomnia and depression are so closely linked, in fact, that if you are experiencing insomnia, you or your doctor should look for signs that you also have depression. If you do have depression, treating it will be a key part of solving your sleep problems.

Anxiety Disorders

Generalized anxiety disorder, panic disorder, post-traumatic stress disorder, and other anxiety disorders often lead to sleep deprivation.

Generalized anxiety disorder is excessive anxiety and worry that are difficult to control and that are causing distress or impairment. A person is considered to have this disorder if the anxiety is associated with at least three of the following symptoms:

- Restlessness; feeling keyed up or on edge
- Being easily fatigued
- Difficulty concentrating or mind going blank
- Irritability
- Muscle tension
- Sleep disturbance

Three-quarters of people with this disorder report that their sleep is disturbed. They have trouble getting to sleep and staying asleep. Some people say they feel sluggish or have "nervous exhaustion" in the morning.

Panic disorder causes sudden, intense anxiety and dread in the absence of circumstances that might normally provoke panic, such as a physical threat. The symptoms include breathlessness, racing heartbeat, choking, chest pain, dry mouth, hot and cold flashes, dizziness, nausea, and fear of losing control or dying. Panic disorders may increase the chance of insomnia, particularly awakening too early. Sufferers often say their sleep is restless, fragmented, or not refreshing. Also, many sufferers have panic attacks during sleep. These attacks usually occur during sleep other than REM sleep, so they do not arise from dreams. Intense, sudden fear and apprehension jolts the sleeper awake. A full-blown panic attack makes it difficult to get back to sleep.

Also associated with sleep problems is post-traumatic stress disorder. This condition can occur when a person witnesses or experiences a life-threatening or terrifying event like a crime, rape, military combat, torture, accident, or serious illness. Initial responses of fear, helplessness, or horror give rise to recurrent and intrusive memories of the event. Insomnia, anxiety, panic attacks, and flashbacks during the sleep period are commonly reported by people who suffer from post-traumatic stress, and about two-thirds experience nightmares, often about their experience.

Dementia

Dementia is an erosion or loss of mental abilities, such as memory, so severe that normal function is seriously impaired or lost altogether. The most common type of dementia is Alzheimer's disease. Although Alzheimer's disease is a devastating illness, it affects only 2 percent to 4 percent of people over age sixty-five.

About 40 percent of people with Alzheimer's disease have significantly disturbed sleep; in fact, disturbed sleep may first alert the family that something is wrong. People with Alzheimer's wake frequently during the night. One serious sleep problem characteristic of dementia is "sundowning," disruptive behavior and agitation before or during the customary sleep time. Sundowning is among the most common reasons that demented patients enter nursing homes. Family caregivers are often able to deal with the cognitive problems associated with dementia, but understandably, when the nighttime calm of the household is disrupted by sundowning, the stress becomes too great.

If You Suspect Your Problem Is a Medical Disorder

If you already know you have one of the above medical problems, you may have been surprised to learn that your sleep problems come with the territory. If your condition improves, your sleep can, too. Often, though, insomnia feeds on itself, and you may need to break the pattern with the techniques recommended for insomnia.

If you have sleep problems but aren't currently being treated for a medical problem, consider the possibility of an underlying physical

＊☾＊☾＊☾＊☾＊☾＊☾＊

Medications That Can Affect Sleep

Some sleep problems are caused not by a medical disorder itself but also by the prescription or nonprescription drugs used to treat it. Sleep disruption can occur either while taking the drug or afterwards during a withdrawal period. If you are taking any medication and are experiencing insomnia, ask your doctor or pharmacist whether insomnia is a known side effect. Unfortunately, sometimes it is necessary to continue a medication even if it does interfere with sleep. But other times, the drug, dose, or timing can be changed. The following drugs are among those known to cause sleep problems.

amphetamines
antidepressants (SSRIs and MAOIs)
antihypertensives
antihistamines (daytime drowsiness, increased difficulty getting to sleep at night)
appetite suppressants
benzodiazepines (rebound insomnia after drug stopped)
caffeine
calcium channel blockers
cholesterol-lowering agents
corticosteroids
levodopa
methysergide
nicotine
oral contraceptives
theophylline
thyroid replacement hormones

cause. Schedule an examination by your doctor. Tell your doctor that you have been having trouble with sleep and mention any symptoms you are experiencing. Sleep problems may actually do you a favor, by being a warning sign of a serious health problem that should be treated.

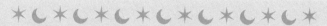

Sleep Problem Questionnaire

Now that you've learned about the various causes of sleep deprivation, these questions will help you clarify the possible sources of your sleep problem. Answer yes or no:

- *Are you sleepy during the day, even though you fall asleep right away when you go to bed and usually sleep through the night without awakening?*
- *Do you sometimes fall asleep during the day without planning to?*
- *Do you sleep longer than usual on weekends or vacations?*
- *When you do sleep longer, do your fatigue and sleepiness go away?*
- *Has your sleepiness lasted at least three months?*
- *Is there no obvious medical or sleep disorder that would account for your sleepiness?*

If you have answered yes to most of these questions, you may be getting insufficient sleep. Chapter 4 will help you figure out how much sleep you need.

- *Do you often have difficulty falling asleep?*
- *During the night, do you awaken frequently or for long periods?*
- *Do you awaken too early and then find that you cannot return to sleep?*
- *Do you feel fatigued or tired during the day?*
- *Does your sleep loss affect your mood or mental performance?*
- *When you can't sleep do you feel afraid, worried, or angry?*

If you've answered yes to any of these questions, you may have insomnia. Chapters 4 and 6 are important for you.

- *Do you go to bed and wake up at varying times from day to day?*
- *Do you have an alcoholic drink before bedtime?*
- *During the day, do you use products that contain nicotine or caffeine?*
- *Do you "try too hard" to fall asleep?*
- *Do you sleep in a bed or room that feels uncomfortable?*
- *Do you worry during the sleep period?*
- *Do you lack a presleep routine?*

If you've answered yes to any of these questions, you may have poor sleep habits. See chapter 5 for details.

- *Do you feel you must take a sleeping pill to go to sleep?*
- *Do you experience withdrawal symptoms if you try to stop taking sleeping pills?*
- *Has your doctor or a sleep specialist recommended sleeping pills, but you've been afraid to try them?*

If you answered yes to any of these questions, you need to learn more about sleeping medications. See chapter 7.

- *Do you experience sleep difficulties or sleepiness as a result of shift work?*
- *Do you experience sleep difficulties or sleepiness when you travel across multiple time zones?*
- *Do you regularly fall asleep and rise much later than you want to?*
- *Do you regularly fall asleep and rise much earlier than you want to?*
- *Are you unable to keep a consistent sleep schedule no matter how hard you try?*

If you answered yes to any of these questions, you may have a circadian rhythm disorder. See chapter 8.

- *Do you snore?*
- *Has anyone ever told you that you have trouble breathing during sleep, or that you stop breathing periodically?*
- *Are you a restless sleeper?*
- *Do you awaken feeling uneasy for no apparent reason?*
- *Do you frequently awaken with a headache?*
- *If you are male, do you have difficulty getting or maintaining an erection?*
- *Do you have high blood pressure or heart disease?*

If you answered yes to any of these questions, you may have sleep apnea or another sleep-related breathing disorder. See chapter 10.

- *Do you regularly have an overwhelming urge to sleep during the day?*
- *Upon falling asleep or waking up, do you experience unusual events, such as seeing things or hearing things that aren't really there?*
- *Upon falling asleep or waking up, do you feel you cannot move your muscles?*
- *Have you ever experienced sudden weakness or a loss of muscle strength, particularly in response to an extreme emotion like anger or laughter?*

If you answered yes to any of these questions, you may have narcolepsy. See chapter 10.

- *Do you experience a "creepy crawly" feeling or other unusual sensation in your lower legs just before going to sleep or upon waking?*
- *Do you often try to "walk off" such sensations?*
- *Have you been told that your legs twitch or jerk while you sleep?*

If you answered yes to any of these questions, you may have restless legs syndrome or periodic limb movement disorder. See chapter 10.

- *Do you grit or grind your teeth during sleep?*
- *Do you talk in your sleep?*
- *Do you walk in your sleep?*
- *Do you eat while you appear to be asleep?*
- *Are you violent in your sleep?*
- *Do you wet your bed?*
- *Do you suffer from nightmares or night terrors?*
- *Do you awaken feeling confused?*

If you answered yes to any of these questions, you may have a parasomnia. See chapter 10.

- *Do you have health problems that affect your sleep?*
- *Do headaches wake you up at night?*
- *Do you have heartburn?*
- *Have you ever had a seizure during sleep?*
- *Does a painful condition awaken you?*

If you answered yes to any of these questions, a medical problem may be interfering with your sleep. See chapter 10 and schedule an appointment with your doctor.

✳ 4 ✳

A Time to Sleep

As a sleep specialist, one of the most common questions that I am asked is, How much sleep do I need? There's no instant answer, as your need for sleep is as individual as you are. In this chapter, you'll learn how to determine your present sleep habits and your actual sleep needs. Then you'll learn how to modify your sleep schedule to promote better sleep. Knowing your personal need for sleep is a key step toward curing sleep deprivation and insomnia.

ON AVERAGE

While sleep averages aren't close enough for our purposes, they're an interesting place to start. The foundation of our current knowledge about sleep need is a study of more than 800,000 people nearly twenty years ago. The study revealed that, on average, most adults between the ages of thirty and sixty-five sleep between seven and nine hours a night.

- More than 40 percent sleep eight to nine hours most nights.
- About 30 percent sleep seven to eight hours.
- One in one thousand sleeps fewer than four hours a night.
- Six in one thousand sleep more than ten hours a night.

When compared to earlier surveys, recent studies have also shown a dramatic reduction in total nightly sleep time over the past century. According to a report by the National Commission on Sleep Disorders, average nightly sleep time has fallen more than 20 percent in the past century, or about two hours a night. Adults are not the only ones whose sleep habits have changed. Around 1900, children between the ages of eight and twelve slept an average of 10.5 hours per night. Teens between the ages of thirteen and seventeen slept about 9.5 hours per night. By 1968, the total nightly sleep time for children and adolescents had dropped by 1.5 hours.

A human need for sleep that evolved over eons cannot change so drastically in just one century. The decreases in sleep time reflect not evolution, but technological and social changes. For example, one thing we're doing instead of sleeping is working. Americans have added approximately 158 hours to their annual work and commuting time— about twenty-six minutes a day—since 1969.

Further evidence of the general trend toward sleep deprivation comes from studies showing that a significant percentage of adults nap when they have the opportunity to do so (e.g., on the weekends) and report daytime sleepiness. Since napping and sleepiness are key signs of insufficient sleep, these findings verify that the hours trimmed from sleep in this century are hours of needed sleep.

Another approach to the question of sleep need was taken in a fourteen-day study of young adults. The study participants reported that they usually slept for about 7.5 hours per day. They were invited to sleep in a laboratory environment without being awakened by alarm clocks or other means. Each young adult was allowed to choose their bedtime and to awaken spontaneously. Over the two weeks, the participants increased their average sleep time to 8.6 hours per day.

Another study of sleep need was performed in two phases. In phase one, time in bed was limited to 8 hours per day. During this phase, the total daily sleep time averaged about 7.4 hours. During the second phase, the participants were allowed to sleep without interruption. They chose their bedtimes and slept until they awoke spontaneously. The subjects who had been sleeping 7.4 hours per night increased their sleep time to an average of 8.9 hours, a whopping 20 percent more.

Such studies provide a broad view of most people's sleep habits and needs. We can use this information to make generalizations about large groups of people, but applying generalizations to an individual is another matter. It's true that on average, people sleep between seven and eight hours a night, but since it is an average, many people sleep less and many people sleep more. Where you fall in the spectrum is based on your own individual habits and needs.

KEEPING A SLEEP LOG

The best way ever developed to reveal sleep patterns is the sleep log. It is a chart on which you keep a daily record of the time you get into bed, the length of time before sleep onset, the number and duration of any awakenings, the time you wake up, the time you get out of bed, and the frequency and duration of naps. The process is simple and easy to learn. But you must make your entries every day, without fail, while your memory is still fresh. Most people make their notes first thing in the morning.

A sleep log will tell you how much sleep you are getting around the clock and how much more sleep you may need. Cross-checks have shown that the information that people enter in their logs is remarkably consistent with the information obtained from more formal and costly sleep-laboratory evaluations. So I strongly recommend that you give the sleep log a try.

ROSEMARY'S SLEEP LOG

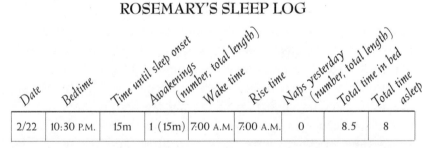

Date	Bedtime	Time until sleep onset	Awakenings (number, total length)	Wake time	Rise time	Naps yesterday (number, total length)	Total time in bed	Total time asleep
2/22	10:30 P.M.	15m	1 (15m)	7:00 A.M.	7:00 A.M.	0	8.5	8

Let's look at an example of a sleep log filled out by Rosemary.

Each night's sleep is recorded on a new line. The advantage of the numeric method is that it gives you columns of numbers that can be used to calculate the total time in bed, total time asleep, and other useful figures.

Rosemary's log shows that she went to bed at 10:30. She fell asleep at about 10:45. During the night, she awakened for about 15 minutes. She then returned to bed and slept without interruption for another 4 hours. She awakened and immediately rose at 7:00 A.M. The summary of this single night is that Rosemary obtained 8 hours of sleep between 10:30 P.M. and 7:00 A.M., interrupted by one brief awakening. This snapshot of a single night provides interesting information about Rosemary's experience on that night; however, it's not as useful as information on several nights. You will get the best results if you record seven to fourteen consecutive days of information, being sure to include information from at least one, but preferably two, weekends.

Most people find it's best to enter information for the preceding night shortly after awakening in the morning, for example at breakfast. Absolutely do not work on completing the log during the sleep period. Estimate the times as best as you can without looking at the clock.

Many people are surprised by the patterns that emerge from their sleep logs. They don't realize they've been spending so little time on sleep or that their schedule varies so much. A sleep log provides not only numerical data but also an overall impression of sleep patterns. The process can be quite illuminating.

On the following page is a blank sleep log for you to copy and fill in.

Analyzing Your Sleep Log

Once you have filled out your sleep log for seven to fourteen days, you can calculate your average bedtime, sleep time, and other important numbers. There's a bit of math involved, but it's pretty basic. Try not to get thrown; follow the steps, stick with it, and soon you'll be calculating your sleep times just like a sleep specialist does. Now grab your calculator, and let's work through a sleep log recorded by Jonathan for ten consecutive days. Like Rosemary's log, Jon's log reveals a typical schedule.

SLEEP LOG

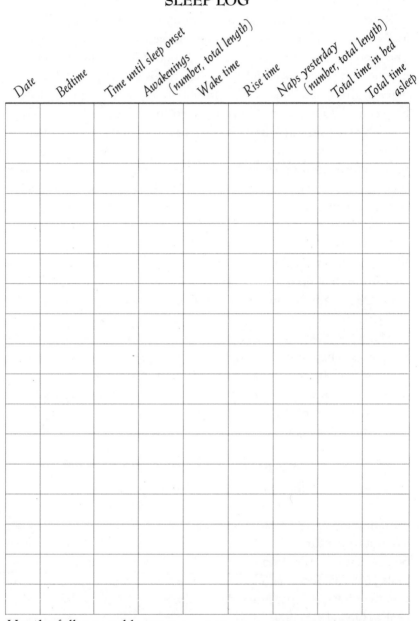

Date	Bedtime	Time until sleep onset	Awakenings (number, total length)	Wake time	Rise time	Naps yesterday (number, total length)	Total time in bed	Total time asleep

Use the following abbreviations: A.M. = morning, P.M. = evening, h = hours, m = minutes. Examples: 7:15 A.M. = 7:15 in the morning; 8h:45m = 8 hours, 45 minutes.

JON'S SLEEP LOG

Date	Bedtime	Time until sleep onset	Awakenings (number, total length)	Wake time	Rise time	Naps yesterday (number, total length)	Total time in bed	Total time asleep
3/1	10:30 P.M.	5m	0	7:30 A.M.	7:30 A.M.	0	9	8.9
3/2	11:30 P.M.	5m	0	8:00 A.M.	8:00 A.M.	0	8.5	8.4
3/3	11:30 P.M.	5m	0	8:00 A.M.	8:00 A.M.	0	8.5	8.4
3/4	10:00 P.M.	10m	0	7:30 A.M.	7:30 A.M.	0	9.5	9.3
3/5	11:00 P.M.	5m	0	7:30 A.M.	7:30 A.M.	0	8.5	8.4
3/6	11:00 P.M.	5m	0	7:30 A.M.	7:30 A.M.	0	8.5	8.4
3/7	11:30 P.M.	5m	1 (30m)	7:30 A.M.	7:30 A.M.	0	8	7.4
3/8	11:30 P.M.	5m	0	7:30 A.M.	7:30 A.M.	0	8	7.9
3/9	10:30 P.M.	5m	0	8:00 A.M.	8:00 A.M.	0	9.5	9.4
3/10	12:30 A.M.	5m	0	8:00 A.M.	8:00 A.M.	0	7.5	7.4

✳︎☾✳︎☾✳︎☾✳︎☾✳︎☾✳︎☾✳︎☾✳︎

Turning Clock Time into Decimal Figures

Before you can do calculations with times, you sometimes need to convert the minutes into decimal figures by dividing them by 60. For example, a bedtime of 10:15 converts to 10.25. A bedtime of 10:45 equals 10.75. To convert back to "clock time," multiply the figure to the right of the decimal point by 60.

Total Time in Bed. Time in bed is the amount of time spent between getting into bed to start the sleep period and getting out of bed for the day. Do not include time spent in bed napping. For each night, convert the time Jon went to bed and the time he got out of bed into decimal figures. He got into bed at 10:30 P.M., or 10.5. He got out of bed at 7:30, or 7.5. Because the bedtime is before 12:00, follow these steps: 12 minus 10.5 plus 7.5 equals 9 hours.

If the bedtime is 12:00 midnight or later, simply subtract the bedtime from the rise time. If the bedtime is between 12:00 and 1:00, count that at the zero hour (for example, 12:15 would be 0.25). A person who goes to bed at 2:15 A.M. and rises at 10:00 A.M. would have a total time in bed of 7.75.

Total Time Asleep. Not all time in bed is spent sleeping. From the total time in bed, subtract any minutes or hours spent awake just after getting into bed, during the night, or just before getting out of bed in the morning.

The log shows that on the first night Jon went to bed at 10:30 and got to sleep at 10:35. He awoke at his normal rising time, 7:30 A.M., with no interruptions. To determine total time asleep, start with the total time in bed (9 hours) and subtract any minutes or hours spent awake at the beginning, end, or middle of the sleep period. In this case, he spent 5 minutes between lights out and sleep and no time awake during the night or upon awakening, so his total sleep time is 9 hours minus .1, or 8.9.

On March 7, when he awoke during the night: 8 hours (total time in bed) minus .1 (time spent falling asleep) minus .5 (awakening during night) equals 7.4 hours spent asleep.

Average Bedtime. Convert all the bedtimes into decimal figures and then add them up. In Jon's case, they add up to 111. Divide by 10 for the average: 11.1. To make the average bedtime easier to read, you have to reconvert the decimals into "clock time," 11:06 P.M.

If Jon had gone to bed at 1:00 A.M. or later, you would have had to use another method to calculate the average bedtime:

1. Convert all bedtimes into decimal figures.
2. Subtract each bedtime earlier than midnight from twelve. Add up the results.

3. Add up all bedtimes later than midnight.
4. Subtract the results of step 2 from the results of step 3.
5. Divide by the number of days to get the average time from midnight. If the answer is a positive number, the bedtime is after midnight. If the answer is a negative number, the bedtime is before midnight; subtract the number you get from midnight.

In the example of Robert that follows, you'd do the following calculation:

- .5 + .5 = 1
- 3.5 + 1.5 + 2.0 + 3.0 + 1.5 + 1.5 + 1.75 + 0 = 14.75
- 14.75 − 1 = 13.75
- 13.75 divided by 10 is 1.375, or 1:23 A.M.

Average Time to Sleep Onset. Now let's calculate Jon's average "sleep latency," the time it takes him to fall asleep. As you can see, Jon falls asleep quickly. Add up the minutes for all the days, divide by 10, and you find that on average, it takes Jon 5.5 minutes to fall asleep at night.

Average Rise Time. We can also calculate Jon's average rise time. Once again, it will be necessary to convert the rise time to minutes (7:30 = 7.5; see box). Then add up all the days and divide by 10. The average rise time is 7.7. Multiply the .7 by 60 to reconvert the figure into "clock time." Jon's average wake-up time is 7:42 A.M.

Average Total Time in Bed. Next, we can calculate Jon's average total time in bed. Add up the column of total times in bed and then get an average by dividing by 10: 8.25, or 10 hours and 15 minutes.

Average Total Time Asleep. Add up the column of total time asleep and divide by 10. Jon's average total nightly sleep time is 8.39, or 8 hours and 23 minutes, and he has no daytime naps.

The Sleepiness Scale

After going through all of these calculations, is it possible to determine Jon's sleep need? Not yet! His sleep log calculations only describe his sleep habits or patterns. To determine if his habits are providing the amount he needs, Jon can ask himself five questions, which I call the "sleepiness scale."

Answer yes or no:

1. Do I experience sluggishness or fatigue at any time during the day?
2. Do I experience sleepiness at any time during the day?
3. Do I have a tendency to doze off or nap?
4. Do I tend to sleep more when given the opportunity?
5. Does my mood, health, or performance during the day seem to be impaired by fatigue or sleepiness?

If Jon's answer to each question is a definite no, it's fair to say that he is getting an adequate amount of sleep at night. But if the answer to *any one* of these questions is yes, it is indeed possible that he is not getting sufficient sleep.

Late to Bed and Early to Rise

Jon was in good shape in the sleep department. He fell asleep quickly, rarely woke during the night, and was averaging 8 hours and 24 minutes of sleep. Indeed, he readily answered no to the five sleepiness questions.

For contrast, let's look at the completed log of someone who was quite a bit sleepier during the day—and until he saw the sleep log, didn't realize why. Robert, a twenty-three-year-old university student in Manhattan, was working through a very difficult basic science curriculum in the hope of attending medical school or graduate school. With his full course load, he studied at least four hours a day outside of class, usually in the late afternoon. When not in class or in the library, Robert had an active social life. He was a loyal fan of team sports, especially basketball and football, which he watched faithfully on TV. He also enjoyed playing basketball occasionally with his buddies. In addition to this very busy academic and recreation schedule, Robert worked two nights a week as a waiter at a local restaurant, which helped make ends meet.

If we look closely at Robert's sleep log, we can see clearly the impact that his busy schedule was having on his life: irregular bedtimes,

ROBERT'S SLEEP LOG

Date	Bedtime	Time until sleep onset	Awakenings (number, total length)	Wake time	Rise time	Naps yesterday (number, total length)	Total time in bed	Total time asleep
10/1	3:30 A.M.	5m	0	7:30 A.M.	7:30 A.M.	1 (30m)	4	3.9
10/2	1:30 A.M.	15m	0	8:00 A.M.	8:00 A.M.	1 (30m)	6.5	6.25
10/3	11:30 P.M.	5m	0	6:30 A.M.	6:30 A.M.	1 (20m)	7	6.9
10/4	2:00 A.M.	10m	0	10:30 A.M.	10:30 A.M.	0	8.5	8.3
10/5	3:00 A.M.	15m	0	10:45 A.M.	10:45 A.M.	0	7.75	7.5
10/6	1:30 A.M.	5m	0	7:30 A.M.	7:30 A.M.	1 (20m)	6	5.9
10/7	1:30 A.M.	5m	0	8:30 A.M.	8:30 A.M.	1 (30m)	7	6.9
10/8	11:30 P.M.	20m	0	6:30 A.M.	6:30 A.M.	0	7	6.17
10/9	1:45 A.M.	5m	0	8:00 A.M.	8:00 A.M.	0	6.25	6.15
10/10	12:00 A.M.	5m	0	8:00 A.M.	8:00 A.M.	1 (30m)	8	7.9

fluctuating rise times, and a slim six to seven hours of sleep per night. For some people, this much sleep might be enough. However, the sleepiness questions revealed daytime fatigue, sleepiness, and inappropriate episodes of sleep, including evening naps. Robert was clearly suffering from insufficient sleep.

Using his log, we can determine the following about Robert's sleep habits:

- Average bedtime, 1:24 A.M.
- Average time until sleep, 9 minutes
- Average rise time, 8:10 A.M.
- Average total time in bed, 6 hours and 48 minutes
- Average total time asleep, 6 hours and 39 minutes

- Average nap time, 16 minutes (averaged over ten days, not just the days he napped)

Robert's bedtimes and rise times were very irregular, and he got up much later on weekends (October 4 and 5) than on weekdays, very likely to compensate for lost sleep during the week. His persistent complaints of fatigue, sleepiness, and inappropriate episodes of sleep during the day pointed directly to insufficient sleep.

DETERMINING *YOUR* SLEEP NEED

Your sleep log will reveal the average number of hours you are sleeping now. The sleepiness scale will reveal whether or not this number of hours is filling your needs. If all your answers were no, you are probably not suffering from sleep deprivation. But if you're reading this book, chances are you had a least one yes. Even one affirmative answer is a potential sign of sleep deprivation.

So how much sleep *should* you be getting? Determining sleep need takes a bit of experimentation, but the sleep log makes this task easier. The simplest approach is to start by going to bed thirty minutes earlier than your *average* bedtime (not the bedtime you'd planned for a particular night) or waking up thirty minutes later than your average wake time. Once you've established this change, keep another log for seven to ten days and retake the sleepiness scale. If you can now answer no to all the questions, you've accomplished your task. If you're still saying yes, sleep deprivation is still present, and I would recommend that you advance your bedtime or move up your wake time by another thirty minutes. Continue until all your responses are a definite no.

If you are allowing yourself more time to sleep but your level of alertness is not improving, you may have an underlying sleep disorder that can't be treated by simply getting more sleep.

Let's look again at Robert's sleep log. We know that he was not getting enough sleep at night and was compensating with evening naps. His average total sleep per day was 6 hours and 27 minutes, and not surprisingly, he reported daytime fatigue. He started by retiring 30 minutes earlier than his average bed time of 1:30 A.M. *every day*. Retiring earlier might seem difficult for Robert; however, he was usually

✶ ☾ ✶ ☾ ✶ ☾ ✶ ☾ ✶ ☾ ✶ ☾ ✶ ☾ ✶

Three Steps to Determine Your Sleep Need and End Sleep Deprivation

1. Use a sleep log to monitor your sleep habits.
2. After ten days, complete the sleepiness scale.
3. If you answer yes to any item on the scale, increase your total daily sleep time gradually in thirty minute increments until all your responses to the sleepiness scale are no.

sitting in his recliner at the end of his day and sometimes dozed off just prior to bedtime. So for him it was a matter of deciding to get out of the recliner, turn off the television, and get into bed one-half hour earlier than usual. Going to bed a half-hour earlier increased Robert's total daily sleep time to 7 hours and 9 minutes, which he recorded on his sleep log. This extra time wasn't enough to improve his fatigue, so we kept extending Robert's sleep time in 30-minute increments until he reported improvement on the sleepiness scale. Robert found that he needed an hour and a half more sleep a night than he had been getting.

GETTING IN RHYTHM

Many people ask me if getting enough sleep is all that counts. Emphatically: *no*. Another very important aspect of sleep is regularity. A regular schedule is essential to sleep for many reasons. For one thing, we are creatures of habit. Having the major components of our daily routines—relationships, meal times, diet, work schedule, bedtime, rise time—in place gives us peace of mind, and peace of mind helps us relax and rest well.

Even more important, establishing a regular pattern reinforces the timing of the body's internal biological clock. In addition to the cycles of sleep stages, another cycle also profoundly affects when we sleep and when we are awake. This cycle is the *circadian rhythm* of sleep

and wakefulness that is tied to the greatest cycle on earth—the end-
lessly dependable rhythm of darkness and light caused by the rotation of the earth.

Our human biological clock runs on a circadian (from the Latin
circa = about, *dian* = day) rhythm that spans about 25.9 hours. Two
twentieth-century German researchers, Jurgen Aschoff and Rutger
Wever, determined the length of the circadian cycle. They isolated
some people in an underground bunker for a month, taking away sunlight, clocks, and other time cues. Each person was allowed to sleep
whenever he wished. Under these conditions, the study participants
had no way of knowing when one day ended and the next began. Remarkably, the results showed that everyone had an internal biological clock that produced a rhythm of sleep and wakefulness, as well as
body temperature, that was slightly longer than one day. The cycle
was 25.9 hours long, so every thirteen days, each person "lost" time
equivalent to one entire day.

The circadian rhythm helps to govern the daily cycle of sleep and
wakefulness, body temperature, metabolic rate, and hormone release.
This rhythm is generated by a small but powerful part of the brain
known as the suprachiasmatic nucleus.

To some people, the discrepancy between this 25.9-hour rhythm
and the 24-hour day suggests that our biological rhythm is imperfect.
Not so! Although the human circadian rhythm runs slightly slower
than 24 hours, it is normally cued to the geophysical day so that our
biological functions (sleeping, waking, burning energy, etc.) can coincide with calendar days. Our cues are taken primarily from exposure to light—one of the human body's most remarkable adaptations
to its environment.

The circadian rhythm is an important modulator of sleep and wakefulness. It is partly this rhythm that governs our natural tendency to
feel sleepy at regular times each day and to stop sleeping at regular
times each day. As you probably know from personal experience, this
rhythm causes two periods of increased sleepiness: one during the night
and the other one during the late afternoon.

Disruption of the circadian rhythm can result in sleep disruption
and sleep deprivation. It can also perpetuate insomnia. For example,
if you habitually lay awake in bed for long periods before falling asleep
for the night and then rise later the next day to compensate for the

lost sleep, it's possible that your circadian rhythm will shift over time. Once this shift occurs, your rhythms of sleeping and waking, body temperature, and hormone release may significantly change. You become more likely to fall asleep later than desired and awaken later than desired each day because the rhythms have all been shifted to a later time. At the other extreme, a person who begins waking up too early, becomes fatigued earlier in the evening, and then retires early can perpetuate early-morning insomnia because the circadian rhythm may shift to an earlier time.

A Regular Rise Time

The best way to get in sync with your circadian rhythm is to establish a regular rise time—the time that you will be out of bed every morning and active. Why rise time instead of bedtime? Because rise time is much easier to manipulate. We can easily use artificial means, such as alarm clocks, to interrupt sleep at a precise, planned time. Planning the onset of sleep at the beginning of the night is neither precise nor dependable.

You can always rise earlier than your regular rise time but avoid getting up later. Ideally, you should vary your rise time by no more than one hour. If your rise time is 7:00 A.M. and you awaken at 6:00 or 6:30 A.M., it's okay to get up and start your day, but you should avoid getting up later than 7:00 A.M. If you find yourself chronically "sleeping in" past 8:00 A.M., consider it a sign that you are not getting enough sleep.

How does this work in practice? A woman named Susan who complained of daytime sleepiness normally rose at 7:00 A.M. on weekdays but slept in until 11:00 A.M. or noon on the weekends. I recommended that Susan establish a regular rise time that she could maintain every day of the week. Since she is employed, Susan had to select a time that conformed to her work schedule, which was the time she currently woke during the week, 7:00 A.M. She then strove to be up at 7:00, or no later than 8:00, no matter what happened the night before.

Setting a rise time may seem inconsistent with earlier recommendations to determine your sleep need and increase your total daily sleep time to meet that need. If you're keeping irregular bedtimes or went to bed too late, shouldn't you stay in bed longer in the morning in order to recover? In some cases of acute sleep loss this may be the answer, but sleeping later is generally not the best response to chronic patterns of sleep loss. The best recommendation—you guessed it—is to keep a regular bed time—one that allows you to obtain sufficient sleep.

The prospect of getting up at 7:00 A.M. on Saturday and Sunday may not sound appealing if you have been in the habit of sleeping late on those mornings, but consider this: Susan will add *ten hours* to her weekend if she's not asleep between 7:00 A.M. and noon. That's more than an average workday at the office! Second, the early morning hours can be the most satisfying part of the day. You can use that time to clear the deck of chores so that by 10:00 A.M. you're ready to enjoy your weekend with a clear conscience. Or you can sit on your deck and watch the sun come up. Or read the paper and work the crossword puzzle without interruptions from the phone or the rest of the family.

A Regular Bedtime

Getting under the covers with the TV remote in hand is not bedtime. Bedtime is the time you get into bed and turn out the lights, ready for sleep. Base your bedtime on the sleep needs revealed by the sleep log and on your chosen rise time:

1. Establish your sleep need.
2. Set the rise time.
3. Work backwards from the rise time to determine the appropriate bedtime.

For example, if your sleep log shows that you need 9.5 hours of sleep per night, and you must rise at 8:30 A.M. to get ready for work, count backwards 9.5 hours from 8:30 A.M. to find your ideal bedtime, which is 11:00 P.M. If you need 7.5 hours of sleep but must rise at 5:00 A.M. to work, count backwards from the rise time to find the ideal bedtime at 9:30 P.M.

People often object to the idea of a regular rise time and regular bedtime. They respond: "I want to go out on the weekends" or "I work late some nights" or "I have a favorite television show that comes on after my bedtime." Some variability is inevitable in everyone's sleep schedule. The goal is not to eliminate variability altogether, but to establish a schedule that will minimize variations most of the time. Then when schedule challenges do arise, you will be better able to deal with the sleep loss and the disruption of timing.

The sleep log and sleepiness scale will help you determine how much variation in sleep schedule you can tolerate. If you can vary your bedtimes and rise times without suffering any noticeable effects of sleep deprivation, then you know that you can tolerate more variability in the schedule. If you begin to vary rise time and bedtime and find that your sleep is disrupted, you begin to experience insomnia, or you suffer effects of sleep deprivation, then you know that you must adhere more closely to your schedule.

SPENDING TOO MUCH TIME IN BED

There really is such a thing as spending too much time in bed, and it can contribute to sleep problems. Some people believe that if they can't sleep, they will benefit from resting in bed. *Wrong!* Nothing replaces sleep, not even bed rest. Spending more time in bed can promote wakefulness in bed, not sleep.

You can determine if you're spending too much time in bed by using the sleep log. Divide the average daily sleep time by the average total time spent in bed (the time from lights out at night to lights on in the morning). The resulting percentage is your "sleep efficiency." If it is less than 85 percent, you are probably spending too much time in bed.

If you spend 460 minutes asleep each day and 480 minutes in bed each day, your efficiency is 96 percent (460 divided by 480). Since this value is above 85 percent, you are spending an appropriate amount of time in bed relative to the amount of time that you spend sleeping. This is a good sleep habit that will help encourage sound and restful sleep. However, if you're sleeping only 380 minutes but spending 540 minutes in bed, your sleep efficiency is 70 percent. You're spending 30 percent of your time in bed lying awake, which is far too much time. Something is amiss in your sleep routine or in your ability to obtain the sleep you need.

If you are older than sixty-five, a sleep efficiency of 75 to 80 percent is probably not a cause for concern. As we get older, it is normal to awaken more frequently and take a bit longer to fall asleep. So a slightly lower sleep efficiency is not a sign of spending too much time in bed.

Sometimes spending long periods of wakefulness in bed can't be avoided, especially if you are in the hospital or are bedridden with an illness at home. In general, however, there are many reasons to try to spend an appropriate amount of time in bed:

- It can be quite frustrating to lay awake in bed for long periods waiting for sleep to come. You may toss and turn or experience other difficulties during these periods of wakefulness.
- If you're not finding it frustrating to lay awake in bed for long periods, you may be trying to withdraw from other life situations or may be depressed. These possibilities are certainly worth examining.
- As we shall discuss in chapter 6 on behavioral treatments for insomnia, spending too much time in bed can reinforce an association between the bed and wakefulness, which itself can contribute to insomnia.
- Spending extremely long periods of time lying awake in bed outside of the usual time reserved for sleep may provide an opportunity to drift in and out of sleep. This behavior can distort the normal rhythm of sleep and result in a pattern of short, fragmented sleep episodes that are interrupted by periods of wakefulness.

If your sleep efficiency is not where it should be, you may benefit from sleep restriction therapy, described in chapter 6.

USING LIGHT TO ALTER YOUR SLEEP PATTERNS

Our circadian rhythms of sleep and wakefulness are governed by light cues. Exposure to light synchronizes the body's internal clock with the planet's cycles of dark and light. For most of us who sleep at night and remain awake during the day, sunlight is a natural cue. We awaken in the morning and our exposure to natural sunlight during our awake hours helps maintain the circadian rhythm. In some cases, exposure to artificial indoor light during the day reinforces the pattern, but in other cases, it disrupts it. Also consider that many people spend the whole day indoors, particularly in the winter.

It is possible to manipulate circadian rhythms by changing exposure to light at key times of the day. One study looked at people who suffered from delayed sleep phase syndrome, chronically falling asleep later than desired and awakening later than desired. They were exposed to light treatment of twenty-five hundred lux for two hours every morning for one week. Subsequently, they were able to fall asleep earlier and were more alert in the morning than a control group exposed to dim light.

Ivy, a recent college graduate, was suffering from delayed sleep phase syndrome. She typically went to bed at 3:00 A.M. and awakened at 11:30 A.M. She had had this sleep schedule for more than two years and could not change it despite her attempts to rise early every day. She had become quite frustrated by her inability to hold a job that started at 9:00 A.M. Although she could usually force herself to rise and get to work on time, she felt sleepy and sluggish all morning. At home, she had difficulty falling asleep earlier than 3:00 A.M., even when she went to bed earlier.

Ivy was not suffering from insomnia, because as long as she went to bed at her prescribed hour, she would fall asleep quickly and stay asleep throughout the night. Ivy had a case of delayed sleep phase syndrome. She and I decided to shift her circadian rhythm of sleep and wakefulness with bright light. We used a commercially available light box that she placed on a desk in her study. This box provided ten thousand lux when she was seated approximately fifteen inches away. Ivy was instructed to rise early every morning and sit next to the light for a brief period. She continued the treatment for about one week, after which she began to notice that she was feeling sleepy earlier than 3:00 A.M. and feeling more alert in the morning hours. With the use of the light and careful management of her sleep and wake schedule, Ivy was able to advance her sleep period by three hours, going to bed at 11:45 P.M. and rising at 8:15 A.M. The early-morning exposure to bright light resulted in earlier bedtimes and earlier rise times.

Exposure to light later in the day has been found to delay the start of sleep and the rise time, which is a desired effect for some people.

Dr. Scott Campbell of the Institute of Chronobiology at the New York Hospital–Cornell Medical Center has conducted studies of elderly individuals who tended to fall asleep early and then awaken before the night is over. He has found that early evening exposure to bright light helps delay sleep onset and promotes later awakenings.

You can use light in many ways to shift or maintain your circadian rhythm of sleep and wakefulness. If you are satisfied with your current sleep schedule, you can use light to reinforce your current sleep/ wake pattern. Awakening each morning and exposing yourself to natural sunlight shortly after getting out of bed will help sustain your natural rhythm. However, if you tend to go to bed later than desired and rise later than desired, you may wish to use light to reset your rhythm. To do this you will need to determine your desired rise time and then get up at that time each morning and immediately expose yourself to light. If, on the other hand, you are becoming sleepy and retiring too early in the evening only to awaken too early the next morning, you may wish to try later afternoon or early evening exposure to bright light.

If you decide to use light to shift your rhythm during the summer, you may find it easiest to use natural sunlight. You could go out for a morning or late afternoon walk or eat your meals while sitting outside. If this exposure to natural light doesn't do the trick, or if it is winter or constantly cloudy, you may elect to use an artificial light source. *Do not use a sun lamp or tanning device for this purpose.* The best artificial light sources for resetting your rhythm are units that are sold commercially for this purpose. These sources provide full-spectrum bright light at an appropriate intensity for resetting your rhythm. To use the box, place it on a table in front of you, just slightly above your eyes, tilting slightly downward toward the table top. You can then read or relax, glancing at the box periodically. The reflected light and the direct light exposure from this procedure should give you ample light. An alternative device is a light visor; worn on your head like a regular cap with a visor, it shines artificial light down into your eyes. Some people like the ease and mobility of the light visor.

Most light boxes provide ten thousand lux of illuminance when used according to the manufacturer's specifications. At this intensity, it is reasonable to begin exposure for thirty minutes, and then adjust your dose of light based on your response. If you notice a positive ef-

A Sign of SAD?

Seasonal affective disorder, commonly called SAD, is a mood disorder related to the seasons of the year. People with the disorder experience low mood or depression in the late fall and then find their mood lifts in the spring. One major contributing factor may be the reduced exposure to natural light in the winter. One feature of SAD is that people start to delay their bedtime and rise times, so that they have a sleep pattern akin to that of delayed sleep phase syndrome. So a delay in sleep phase can be a warning sign of SAD. If you feel you may have this disorder, see your physician. Light treatment is often very effective.

fect within one or two weeks, you may want to discontinue the treatment to determine if the results can be sustained without the light. If you have no response during this time period, you can increase the dosing in fifteen-minute increments until you achieve a response, provided that you have no adverse reactions to the light, particularly irritated eyes. People with bipolar or manic-depressive disorder should use a light with caution as it can cause agitation or elevated mood. Since bright light treatment has obvious biological effects and some (albeit minimal) risks, you should consult with your physician before initiating treatment with an artificial light source. It is also a good idea to have an eye examination before beginning, as the treatment is not recommended for people with retinal problems, glaucoma, or cataracts.

NAPPING

Napping is common in many cultures, including our own. According to Dr. David Dinges at the University of Pennsylvania, early studies revealed that 39 percent of adults (ages nineteen to fifty-five) in the United States never napped, 33 percent napped at least once a week, and 11 percent napped four or more times a week. More recent research completed by Dr. Dinges and his colleagues has found that 80 percent of adults nap at least once a week, with an average nap of one hour and thirteen minutes.

The quality of sleep obtained in a nap can be just as good as night-time sleep, so naps can benefit people who can't get all the sleep they need in one block. You probably won't be missing out on any sleep components by using a nap strategy. However, some naps are a sign of chronic sleep deprivation. This *compensatory napping* is an attempt to replace, in full or in part, the sleep lost at night. Studies of compensatory napping have shown a relationship between the amount of sleep lost and the amount of nap time you need to recover. The less sleep you have obtained, the more nap time you require to restore alertness and level of functioning.

Whether such naps are good or bad, harmful or helpful, depends upon you and your lifestyle. Naps are a problem when they are un-planned—often spontaneous—responses to sleep deprivation. These naps occur in classrooms, in meetings, at the theater, or even while out with friends. Because they occur in an inappropriate context, they are usually not refreshing, comfortable, or adequate to satisfy the sleep deficit. Also, the period of sleepiness preceding such naps can be quite dangerous if you are engaged in an important or hazardous activity, such as operating machinery or driving.

Todd, a middle-aged assembly worker, wouldn't have considered driving while feeling fatigued, but he never guessed that sleepiness on his job could be dangerous. He sat right next to a moving assembly line and inspected parts as they passed his work station. During each shift, the line was stopped for fifteen to twenty minutes for adjustments to the machinery. Todd regularly used these breaks to drift off to sleep, literally napping with his head and hands on the assembly line. He sustained minor injuries more than once when the line started abruptly. One evening, he awakened to find his clothing lodged in the moving parts. He was cut and bruised before he could get free.

Although most people are not in such obviously hazardous situations, many of us move routinely in and out of everyday situations that are risk free only if we remain alert and awake. All the following stories are true:

- A babysitter minding small children stretched out on the sofa to rest her feet for a few minutes. She woke to find the house in flames.
- After several hours of predawn hunting, two young men lay

down to rest in the bed of a railroad track (a dangerous habit of hunters in some areas of the country) and immediately fell fast asleep. They weren't awakened by the rumble of an approaching train until it was too late.

- An exhausted sales executive got into the family pool alone around ten P.M. He rested his head on a flotation device. Hours later, he awakened still in the pool, and very fortunate not to have drowned.

Clearly, unplanned naps can be dangerous.

In addition, naps can make it difficult for some people to sleep at night by regularly filling part of the sleep need. Instead of getting eight hours of sleep in one consolidated block, the person may get only six hours at night and two hours from naps. Repeated over time, this pattern can become so ingrained that any attempt to reverse it by going to bed earlier is met with frustration.

If you want to take a planned nap, reserve a time. Then ease the transition to sleep by going some place dark, quiet, and cool and wearing comfortable clothing. Avoid caffeine, nicotine, and exercise before a nap. Following the same good sleep habits you follow at night

Sleep Inertia

Have you ever awakened from a nap feeling like your arms and legs were made of lead, your vision was bobbing like a keg in a tide, and your brain couldn't pull out of one track? This phenomenon is known as sleep inertia. With sleep inertia, your performance following a nap is actually worse than it was before the nap. This decrease normally lasts less than a half hour, but it can be dangerous to do anything that requires alertness and coordination, including something as simple as walking down stairs or carrying boiling water to a teacup. If you awaken to this condition, exercise great caution. Give yourself several minutes for the effects of sleep inertia to wear off before driving, operating machinery, or engaging in any hazardous activity. The cause of sleep inertia is unknown, although it may be caused by naps that are too short to fill the sleep debt. It could also mean that the sleeper has been awakened from a deep stage of sleep.

will help you get the most from a nap. If you take these steps and still cannot sleep during the day, you may not need the nap or your biological rhythm may not favor daytime naps.

Good Naps

Though unplanned naps and compensatory napping can cause problems, planned naps can be very beneficial. In fact, recent research suggests that scheduled naps are one of the best ways to recover from occasional sleep loss. If you can't meet your daily sleep quota on a particular night, a scheduled nap the next day may be exactly the right answer. For example, consider the nurse who is asked to work a second shift one evening, or the retiree who stays out late one night to socialize with friends. Either might try to recover from sleep deprivation by sleeping late the next morning or going to bed earlier the next night—but a planned nap offers a third and probably the best way to recover from the sleep loss.

How long should your nap be if you're trying to recover from sleep deprivation? There's no easy answer. Sometimes you'll need to recover every minute of lost sleep to feel refreshed and restored. At other times, even a brief nap will provide tremendous rejuvenation. Keep in mind, however, that consistently obtaining less than one's sleep quota and then trying to recover by catching a brief nap during the day does not make up for all of the lost sleep, and over time, can result in chronic sleep deprivation.

There are a multitude of situations in which you can use a scheduled nap to recover from sleep loss. Some such naps can be planned far in advance; for example, if you anticipate spending a late night out next weekend, you could schedule a nap for the following day. Naps can also be planned on short notice. An automobile driver who becomes sleepy at the wheel as a result of insufficient sleep can pull over to nap for a short period, possibly preventing a fatigue-related accident. This practice is not as safe as it once was, so if you do nap in your car, it's absolutely imperative that you choose a safe place to park, perhaps at a gas station or a busy rest stop. I myself regularly use a brief nap to avoid driver fatigue. I have a long drive home at the end of my day. So if I'm feeling a bit sleepy, I take a twenty-minute nap in my office before starting my journey. This way, I am better prepared to enjoy the trip, without worrying about my safety on the road.

The value of planned napping has been proven in several studies. Researchers have found that napping really does improve alertness after nighttime sleep deprivation. The results were the same in both laboratory work and the subjective reports that people provide in sleep log studies.

Mood and performance have also been found to improve following naps, although some studies show only a bit of improvement, others more. In the 1970s, J.M. Taub and his colleagues conducted several studies of performance and napping. They found that performance on a reaction-time task improved significantly following naps that were thirty minutes or 120 minutes long, with no difference between the long and short naps. Taub and his colleagues also found that 120-minute nap periods taken in the morning or in the evening equally improved performance on reaction time and memory tests and that a ninety-minute afternoon nap improved reaction time, short-term memory, and vigilance. These benefits lasted several hours. Another study showed that 96 percent of shift workers had a very positive attitude toward night-shift napping, most believing that it increased performance and improved safety on the job.

Naps can also be used to help someone recover from chronic sleep loss at night. For example, a worker who usually works the day shift but who frequently is asked to stay and work additional hours during the late shift, or a new mother who is up several times per night with her baby, may benefit from scheduled naps that help them to recover from sleep loss at night. This is an excellent way to take advantage of

Cockpit Napping

A NASA study revealed that many air crew members were sleepy during flight. When conditions permitted, 11 percent napped for an average of forty-six minutes. Researchers found that planned naps in the cockpit can help reduce the sleepiness or unplanned napping that can impair performance during flight. The Federal Aviation Administration is considering how to integrate napping into the current regulations, and several airlines have already implemented planned cockpit rest based on this research.

★☾★☾★☾★☾★☾★☾★

Sleep and Culture

Although biological processes underlie the timing of sleep, a society's activities and culture also play a role. It is no coincidence that over time, sleep evolved to occur at night when darkness hampered essential functions such as travel, planting, harvesting, hunting, and commerce. Night also is a time when accidents, injuries, or attack by prey are more likely—in primeval times as well as today's urban jungle. So in our society, and in most others, people sleep for one long time at night, with perhaps a nap.

In contrast, members of the Temiars tribe in Indonesia and the Ibans in Sarawak sleep about four hours a night and then nap many times during the day. This schedule, which is called polyphasic, may seem impractical to us, but it is organized around the tribe's cultural norms and schedules of daily activity. In many hot climates, a midday siesta is the cultural norm, allowing everyone to rest in the hottest part of the day.

Behind sleep, as behind all our other habits and activities, lie both nature and nurture. Perhaps some day, every workplace will build in an afternoon siesta. Anyway, it's worth hoping for!

napping. You can awaken refreshed and feeling better for the balance of your day.

You can also use napping as a preventive measure, in advance of anticipated sleep loss. A study showed that night-shift workers who took a two-hour nap before coming to work performed better when tested later in the work shift. Another study found that a brief nap during a fifty-six-hour extended work day improved reaction time and cognitive performance. Interestingly, in such studies participants have not always rated their sleepiness and mood as better following naps, yet they performed considerably better.

In most workplaces, productivity falls in midafternoon, when inner clocks are calling for a nap for an hour or so. The copiers are winking, the machines are blinking, phones are in hand, and heads are nodding, but the entire place may be on automatic pilot while passing through the fog of midafternoon slump. This behavior isn't laziness or goofing off, and it's not fun. Each body fiber demands sleep, but the workplace will not allow it.

If you strongly experience this dip, try to figure out a way to take a brief nap. Use your biological rhythm to your advantage by letting it help you take a wonderfully refreshing nap. Some executives are known to take a regular afternoon "power nap," at which time they shut the office door, dim the lights, and recline in their chair for fifteen minutes of sleep. They awaken feeling refreshed and more alert, and can perform better. Taking a nap break can improve performance and productivity.

Athletes and people in other challenging settings have also used power naps effectively.

* 5 *

Ten Tips for a
Good Night

Some people do all the right things—keep a regular sleep schedule, allow themselves adequate opportunities for sleep—but night after night just can't get to sleep. Or they wake up again and again during the night. By the time I see them, they have full-blown insomnia. Many are frustrated because they're getting enough sleep in the course of a twenty-four-hour day, but the sleep is neither restful nor refreshing. Working together, we often find the solution in a change in sleep habits, particularly the activities before going to bed. In fact, you can count the key sleep habits on each of your fingers. This chapter tells how you can put the ten tips for a good night to work for you.

You don't have to take my word on the value of these tips. They're advocated by most sleep professionals. You may have seen some of these tips in magazines, newspapers, or journals. You may have even tried some, and perhaps they didn't work. Trust me on this: They're worth another try. For one thing, now you're better educated about your sleep habits and sleep needs. You've embarked on a program to correct your sleep problems, and perhaps you are managing your sleep in new ways. (If you have not yet worked through the preceding chapters, go back and do so before trying these tips.) Possibly in the past you weren't prepared to stay with a method long enough for it to work.

The 1-3 Rule

- *Make no more than 3 changes in your sleep habits at 1 time. A change is any one aspect of a tip, not everything covered under that tip. (For example, replacing your mattress, which is part of tip 1, counts as one change.)*
- *Stick with any change that you make for at least 3 weeks before deciding whether or not it is helping.*

You may have tried too many different things at once. The problem then was not the tip, but the approach. I have seen many people make dramatic progress because we were able to implement these tips into an overall treatment program. To structure a program for yourself, follow the 1–3 Rule above.

Decide what to work on first. As you read the chapter, you may note that you drink several cups of caffeinated coffee a day, are a big fan of midnight raids on the refrigerator, and often lie awake with the worries of the day racing through your brain. Choose whichever behavior seems to be the greatest or most obvious source of your problems. Or if you feel you need to build up to the hardest problems, choose one that seems easy and work on it first. Some people like to tackle the hardest change first, to get it out of the way.

After you make a change in your sleep habits, use a sleep log to determine whether your sleep has improved, and how much. Keep a log daily throughout the time that you are working on your sleep habits. Complete the sleep log calculations to determine your improvement. If the improvement is satisfactory, you may want to make the changes a permanent part of your life. If improvement is not satisfactory after three weeks, try a different tip. Evaluate any further changes with a sleep log.

If you make as many changes to your sleep habits as you can, but your sleep doesn't improve significantly, you may wish to pursue a behavioral treatment for insomnia (the next chapter). Also, your problem may be a sleep disorder or medical problem.

✴ ☾ ✴ ☾ ✴ ☾ ✴ ☾ ✴ ☾ ✴ ☾ ✴ ☾ ✴

Ten Tips for a Good Night of Sleep

1. Create a comfortable sleep environment.
2. Don't go to bed stuffed or starving.
3. Get some exercise.
4. Cut out the night cap.
5. Stop smoking.
6. Drink decaffeinated beverages.
7. Check your medications.
8. Leave your worries behind.
9. Establish a helpful presleep routine.
10. Don't try too hard to go to sleep.

TIP 1. CREATE A COMFORTABLE SLEEP ENVIRONMENT

Consider your bed, your pillow, and the levels of light, temperature, and noise in your sleeping place. Are they conducive to a good night's sleep?

Your Bed

As Goldilocks said, the bed shouldn't be too hard or too soft—you need one that is *just right* for you. If your mattress is lumpy or worn, invest in a new one. It will pay years of dividends in restorative sleep.

When you make a purchase, the first thing to consider is the size of the bed. You want to make sure that your bed is large enough to provide ample sleeping surface, especially if you are tall or large. If you are sleeping with a spouse or partner, each person needs enough space to rest comfortably and move freely during sleep without disturbing the other.

Your next consideration is the firmness of the mattress, which is a matter of personal taste and comfort. Many of us find it embarrassing to lie down while a salesman looks on, but there's no other way to choose the right mattress. Stretch out, roll over, lay on your side, and bounce around until you're sure you've got the right one. People with back pain or arthritis may be more comfortable on a firm mattress. If you need firmness but love lush comfort, too, you can add a separate foam or quilted pad, available in the bedding department of most department stores, to the top of the mattress. Once you own the mattress of your dreams, remember to turn it periodically and sleep on the other side, so it will last longer and stay fresher.

The foundation that goes under your mattress is as important as the mattress. Be sure to look closely at what you're getting. Press the palm of your hand into the foundation to see if what you're looking at is a *box spring* (which is what most of us think we're getting) with springs or a tensile wire construction or a *box* (a wooden frame without springs).

If your present mattress has begun to sag in the middle but is otherwise in good condition, you might add a back board—a piece of half-inch or three-quarter-inch plywood, or even a piece of firm plastic—between the mattress and box spring. Another way to prevent or repair a sag in your mattress is to add three to five wooden slats, cut to fit *snugly* between the side rails. Placed under the box spring and mattress, the slats will add support, especially on a queen-size or king frame.

Your Pillow

Even if your mattress and foundation are perfect, you may still have a hard time getting to sleep if your pillow isn't right for you. Your pillow should have the right size, contour, and softness for your sleeping style. Do you prefer to put your back, head, and neck on a large pillow? Or do you sleep with only your head on the pillow? Either position is fine (unless you have reflux or apnea, which tend to be worse when you sleep on your back), but the type of pillow you need will differ. Soft pillows are often good for stomach sleepers, medium pillows for back sleepers, and firm pillows for side sleepers. If you have several pillows, you can create the most comfortable position for your head and neck on any night. If you have back or neck pain during the sleep period or when you awaken, a contour pillow may minimize strain during the night.

Don't forget to consider the content of the pillow, which may be manufactured materials, duck feathers, or goose down. Manufactured materials are stiffer and provide firmer support, while natural materials tend to be softer and more pliable. Feathers are firmer than down. Some people are allergic to down or feathers; if you suffer from itching, burning eyes at night, your pillow may be the problem.

Some of my patients ask whether a hospital bed would help them. The advantage, of course, is that you can elevate your head or feet. Others inquire about special supports, such as wedge-shaped pillows to elevate the head or knees. All of these options are a matter of personal comfort, taste, and budget. Elevating your head can reduce sinus pressure, can reduce orthopnea (breathing difficulties that become worse when you lie down; this is associated with obesity or breathing disorders), and by the force of gravity, can help prevent stomach acids from washing up into the esophagus and causing heartburn or acid reflux. If your feet or ankles swell during the night, try sleeping with your feet elevated. This position relieves discomfort in the legs and feet by reducing the pooling of fluid and blood. However, people with osteoarthritis or rheumatoid arthritis affecting the knees should not prop up their knees all night; while this may provide temporary comfort, very painful muscle and tendon contractions will happen when they have to stand or stretch the leg.

If you recently ended a relationship or lost a spouse or partner and are finding it difficult to sleep alone, you may rest better with a "body pillow," a long, fluffy pillow that plumps the vacant side of the bed. This type of pillow is also a great support for people who have arthritis or other pain in many joints.

While you're focused on your bed and pillow, inspect your sheets, blankets, and comforters. Make sure your sheets feel good against your skin. If you replace sheets, look for those with high thread counts, which are softer than those with lower counts. If you purchase sheets made of a blend of cotton and polyester, look for a higher content of cotton and a lower content of polyester (at least 60 percent cotton, 40 percent polyester). Blend fabrics with a high amount of polyester tend to be hot.

Room Temperature

Temperature extremes—too hot or too cold—can be very disruptive to sleep. Most people sleep best when their bedroom is slightly cool. During winter, you will save energy and enhance your sleep by turning down the thermostat a little at bedtime and using blankets or a nice comforter to get cozy and warm in bed. In really chilly conditions, such as when the furnace breaks down, a sleeping cap and socks on your feet will warm things up. During the summer months, a room air conditioner or central air can be a lifesaver—literally, in some cases—by maintaining a comfortable room temperature.

One reason a cooler bedtime environment is desirable is that your body cools down during sleep. The core body temperature, deep inside, drops to its lowest point during sleep. Sleeping in a slightly cool environment complements the natural drop in body temperature.

An electric blanket may allow you to sleep in a cool environment during the winter. You will naturally adjust your need for the blanket during sleep by covering up less or more of your body. An electric blanket can also be a good way to combat cold feet; wearing socks is another solution.

Humidity

Sometimes it's not only the heat that disrupts sleep but also the humidity. If humidity is too high, the best way to reduce it is a central or room air conditioner.

Dry air is even more disruptive to your health and sleep than humid air. You may wake up with a dry or sore throat, dry nasal passages, or nosebleed. Your skin can also become dry. If your home is dry during the winter months, try a humidifier. Make sure you change the water every day and clean the machine regularly according to the directions.

Air Circulation

For many people, nothing is more conducive to sleep than a gentle breeze billowing the curtains at the windows. Of course, it is a law of the universe that those who love a breeze will mate only with those who must sleep with the windows shut.

If you can't get a breeze by opening a window, a ceiling or floor fan or an air conditioner can help. In addition to helping the body cool down, movement of air prevents room air from becoming stale or stuffy.

Darkness

Most people sleep best when their sleep environment is very or completely dark. If you sleep in a room with windows, especially those that have full exposure to the morning sun, you may have to make a few simple changes. Window shades or lined drapes (or both) are usually sufficient to darken a room. If even a small amount of sunlight, moonlight, or street-lamp light disturbs you, you may wish to purchase special blackout shades that totally cover the window surface. Another alternative is eyeshades, which are effective, economical, and available at your pharmacy.

Before you take steps to further darken your sleep environment, remember that exposure to bright light upon awakening in the morning is an important cue for your circadian rhythm. Exposure to light in the morning can be uplifting and energizing. So if you tend to rise shortly after dawn, you may find it highly desirable to allow morning sunlight to enter your room. This way you begin to get the full effect of the sun at the earliest possible moment. On the other hand, if you have to protect yourself against light in the evening (such as street lights) while you are trying to sleep or you are trying to sleep after the sun has risen, you may find that taking steps to darken your bedroom will be very helpful.

Noise

Noise pollution is less easily managed than some other aspects of your sleep environment. In big cities, traffic, sirens, car alarms, and aircraft noises generate a continuous cacophony that can disturb sleep. Even if we learn to tune out the sounds that surround us, our bodies still respond to each noise.

An auditory threshhold study showed that people become more sensitive to such noise pollution as they grow older. For several nights in a sleep lab, people were exposed to various sounds to study the depth of the various levels of their sleep. An unexpected finding was that after several nights, the younger people became used to the sounds, so they had to be louder to awaken them. Older people, on the other hand, became more likely to be awakened by the same level of sound. Younger people became habituated to sounds, but older people became sensitized. No wonder older people are more likely to complain that noises disrupt their sleep. For them, it is especially important to protect the sleep environment from extraneous noises. But at any age, noise can disrupt both our nights and our days.

The room that you sleep in should be insulated as much as possible from outside noise. Good windows can make a big difference. If noise levels are particularly high in your area (e.g., you live in a big-city apartment), installing double-pane windows can significantly reduce noise. Curtains or drapes, and carpets or rugs, absorb some sound.

If all else fails, try ear plugs. Several types are available from your pharmacist. Most comfortable and effective when sleeping are the small, cylinder-shaped, foam plugs that you roll between your fingers and then insert into the ear canal or the small, waxlike insert that you mold to fit the shape of your ear and press in tightly. Both types fit inside the ear and are not dislodged by head movements during sleep. They also are so soft that they will not awaken you or cause pain if you lie on them the wrong way.

While sudden noises can disrupt sleep, certain low, continuous noises may actually help sleep. Such sounds, called "white noise," mask other noises. You may be surrounded by white noise without being conscious of it: the hum of the washing machine, the whir of a fan overhead, the singing of peepers in the yard. Some people find that white noise is comforting and lulls them to sleep. In fact, white noise is so effective that a commercial product has been created to produce it. This device raises the level of background white noise, making it less likely that sleep will be disrupted by any sudden sounds.

There are more complex sounds that can either help or harm sleep. Some people report that a sound-generating machine that simulates raindrops or waterfalls or tape-recorded soft music is quite conducive to sleep. However, people who use such devices often can't sleep unless the devices are on. If the device goes off, the sleeper may abruptly awaken. To avoid such dependence, I suggest you put the device on a timer so it turns off automatically shortly after you've fallen asleep. Many sleep specialists think that TV and radio can disrupt sleep if they are left on through the sleep period; these are not the best choices of white noise.

Other Environmental Factors

Besides noise, temperature, and your comfy pillow, a few other issues are also related to your sleep environment—some unique to you. The movements of a pet, a drippy faucet, an offensive odor, or a tossing bed partner can all be disturbing. Don't passively accept your environment as is and then struggle to sleep in it. Change it for the better.

✶☾✶☾✶☾✶☾✶☾✶☾✶

Only for Sleep

As much as possible, use your sleep environment only for sleep. If you catch up on work or pay bills in your bedroom, you will associate the room with tension—not the most conducive mood for sleep. Other activities like sewing, exercising, or watching television also won't put you in the right frame of mind.

So take activities other than sleep out of the bed and the bedroom. If you can, move the computer, desk, TV, sewing machine, or exercise equipment somewhere else. If space limitations make this change impossible, think creatively about how you might isolate the sleep area. Here are a few ideas.

- Import stores—those places that carry lots of wicker, bamboo, and decorative items—usually have inexpensive folding screens that not only will do the job but also may add interest to your decor.
- Another trick is to move the bed so that the headboard is at the center of the room and the foot board is a couple of feet from the wall. This is especially appealing if it positions you for a nice view out of a bedroom window when you awaken in the morning. Add a bookcase or table with plants behind the headboard, and you have the elements of a spread in a decorating magazine.
- Back in history, when the bed was often in the main room of the house, it was often surrounded with bed curtains. An easy way to create these is to install six large hooks (available in your hardware store—the type with toggle bolts will be needed for heavy duty) on the ceiling about an inch outside the outlines of your bed—one at each corner and one halfway along each side. Hang inexpensive brass curtain rods from the hooks. Use attractive sheets, curtain panels (eighty-one-inch length), or fabric for curtains. Hang them from the rods using brass "pinch" drapery rings.

TIP 2. DON'T GO TO BED
STUFFED OR STARVING

Hunger pangs are uncomfortable and make it hard to fall asleep. On the other hand, being too full can cause stomach distention, indigestion, gas, or cramping. Hunger or fullness can prevent you from falling asleep and can awaken you during the night. If you feel hungry around bedtime, have a light snack, preferably thirty minutes or more before lights out.

Late-Night Snacks

When you're rummaging around in the kitchen for a snack before bedtime, what should you be looking for? Perhaps the food you're craving is exactly what you should eat—but not if you're craving two cans of sardines with a sliced onion on bread and a couple of colas. The first consideration is to avoid foods that are hard to digest—like those sardines and onions. Don't eat foods that are spicy or oily or have given you problems in the past. Heartburn and acid reflux can really interrupt a night of sleep.

There's a lot of talk in the sleep community about whether certain foods are more conducive to sleep than others. Some experts recommend a high-carbohydrate food (such as bread or pasta) and others a protein (such as meat or a glass of milk). Bowl of cereal and milk, anyone?

You may also have heard that foods high in tryptophan, such as milk, turkey, or meat, may promote sleep. Tryptophan is a precursor to the neurotransmitter serotonin, which helps regulate sleep. While this theory is appealing, I know of no evidence to suggest that tryptophan obtained from foods helps bring sleep. If you have a glass of milk before bed and find it helpful, the reason is probably something other than the tryptophan, perhaps even psychological factors.

A modest sweet snack before bedtime is fine, but too much sugar may increase your energy level and make sleeping more difficult.

Besides making sleep more comfortable, eating a small snack rather than a bedtime feast will also help you keep your weight at a healthy level. While you're asleep, your metabolism falls to its lowest point of the day, making it less likely that you'll burn off extra calories. So, if you crave chocolate-chip cookies and milk, go for a *small* portion of cookies and a *modest* amount of milk. Seal up the cookie bag and put it back in the cabinet before you sit down to your snack, cutting off any temptation to eat the whole bag. Calories add up quickly. A late-night snack of vegetables or fruit is much lower in calories than a sandwich of cold cuts and Swiss cheese, which is lower in calories than other treats such as ice cream, baked goods, or nuts.

Fluids

Limit your fluids at bedtime. If you awaken frequently to urinate during the sleep period, be particularly careful to avoid a large amount of fluids. If you limit fluids but still awaken to urinate, eating something salty, such as a couple of saltine crackers, before bed may help you to retain a little more fluid (assuming you aren't on a sodium-restricted diet). If adjusting your fluid intake at night doesn't resolve the situation, consult your physician. Frequent urination can be a sign of diabetes, urinary tract infection, prostate enlargement, or other health problems.

Midsleep Snacks

Do you wake up in the middle of the night and eat a snack? You'd be surprised how many people do. A trip to the kitchen may satisfy you and allow you to return to sleep more easily. But if you're doing this regularly, it could be a problem. Repeated nightly awakenings for the purpose of eating can prime you to wake up in the middle of the night, and your body will hold sleep ransom until you eat. Before you know it, this pattern will be going on night after night after night.

There are several ways to deal with this problem. One is to stop all eating between bedtime and the time you rise in the morning. Of course, this restriction will be difficult for the first few days, but your body will readjust to the absence of food during the night and the awakenings will stop.

If you can't discontinue eating at night altogether, try gradually reducing the portion or calories until the nighttime eating episodes are eliminated. You'll do better with this approach if you prepare a tray of appropriate food for your midsleep snack in the evening before you go to bed.

Night eating may be a sign that you are not eating enough during the day. If you're deliberately holding down your daytime calorie intake—for example, for weight control—look out for a rebound at night. The calories you consume in a bedtime snack or midsleep meal can easily cancel out an entire day of self-control. It would be better to allow yourself a little more food during the day.

Eating Problems and Sleep

During my years as a fellow at the Westchester Division of the New York Hospital–Cornell Medical Center, I worked with people, mostly young women, who had eating disorders such as anorexia nervosa and bulimia. Many came or were brought to the hospital because they were dangerously underweight and seriously ill from poor nutrition. Many also had severely disturbed sleep. Indeed, research has shown that people who have anorexia nervosa or bulimia and are significantly underweight tend to sleep less than normal, healthy people sleep. Because of the more urgent nutrition problems that require immediate medical or psychiatric attention, the sleep problem is not always identified as a treatment issue, but it also should be addressed.

Another eating problem, obesity, significantly increases the risk of sleep-related breathing disorders, such as sleep apnea, and other medical problems that can disturb sleep.

A sleep disorder recently described by Dr. Carlos Schenck in Minnesota causes people to awaken during the night to eat, but blots out any memory of the snack. People with this disorder eat while they are sleepwalking! Sometimes they consume food, but other times they eat things like raw meat, cat food, or a family-size jar of mayonnaise. One woman even munched on a scouring pad. Typically, these people have little or no memory of the eating binge, so they learn about their nighttime escapades by witnessing the dirty dishes, empty wrappers, leftovers, or stains and soils. A woman who had gorged herself with peanut butter and bread realized that she had done so only because she woke with smears of peanut butter on' her face, arms, and knees. If you suspect that you fit this pattern, you should consult with a sleep specialist.

TIP 3. GET SOME EXERCISE

Whether or not you exercise, you know that it's good for your health. But I bet you didn't know that it can enhance sleep. Exercise does so because it temporarily raises body temperature (a few tenths of a degree centigrade), which adds momentum to the normal fall in body temperature with sleep. Exercise also alleviates physical and mental stress and can help prevent or improve a variety of medical disorders that affect sleep, from arthritis to heart disease. Exercise even changes the architecture of sleep; physically fit people who exercise have a temporary increase in delta (deep) sleep.

Contrary to popular belief, exercise doesn't help you sleep by making your body tired. People who have trouble sleeping aren't helped even when they are physically exhausted. Consider that people who spend their vacations resting on the beach or on a cabin porch often sleep well at night. Though they are temporarily sedentary and are spending their days relaxing, they may well sleep much better than at home.

People who are sedentary most of the time, though, may have difficulty with sleep because the line is blurred between the activity of wakefulness and the activities of the sleep period. People who are chronically sedentary may also have a medical or psychiatric problem that is causing poor sleep.

The kind of exercise that helps with sleep is aerobic exercise, vigorous physical activity, and movement over a sufficient period. Examples are jogging, swimming, rowing, and bicycling. If you exercise indoors, you can get the same effect with a stair-stepper, stationary bicycle, or rowing machine. Twenty or thirty minutes a day is all you'll need to improve your cardiovascular fitness and the quality of your sleep. Non-aerobic exercise (like weight training or stretching) has not been shown to improve sleep.

The timing of your exercise is just as important as the type of exercise. Exercising in the late afternoon or early evening is best. Exercising early in the day is not likely to affect sleep. Exercising *right* before bedtime, though, is counterproductive. It increases alertness, which makes it more difficult to fall asleep and stay asleep. Heavy exercise just before sleep actually reduces delta sleep.

What about Sex?

Every now and then, usually when I am lecturing to a large group and feeling just a bit self-conscious, someone in the audience asks if sexual activity constitutes an appropriate presleep exercise. This always gets a good laugh.

The answer is, although I wouldn't consider sexual activity an exercise, it can influence sleep quality. In Western cultures, sexual ac-

A Nice Warm Bath

Since exercise helps because it raises body temperature, some researchers have investigated whether passive body heating like a warm bath also enhances sleep. These studies have shown that a warm bath before bedtime can significantly improve the ability to fall asleep and stay asleep. A warm shower will probably work, too, but only immersion in a bath has been tested.

tivity is associated with bed and usually takes place just before the beginning of the sleep period. Since orgasm is commonly followed by relaxation, it seems logical that it would ease the way to sleep. This notion has been supported by studies of lower animals, which fall asleep more rapidly following sexual stimulation. However, research performed with humans hasn't revealed any consistent improvement in sleep following sexual activity. For some people, sexual activity can cause hyperarousal. (If you have ever had a mate who got up from your bed to wax the floors, cut the lawn, or hang wallpaper in the bathroom, now you know it wasn't something you said.) People who respond this way to sex may sleep better if they have sex in the morning. Also, under some circumstances, for some people sexual activity can cause anxiety or frustration. These emotions can prolong the time it takes to fall asleep.

Will sexual activity in bed diminish the association between the bed and sleep? For most people, no, but for some, yes. If you feel this particular shoe fits, try engaging in sex outside of your bedroom. One gentleman I counseled reported that this recommendation not only marginally improved his insomnia but also dramatically spiced up his sex life!

TIP 4. CUT OUT THE NIGHT CAP

Because alcohol is a powerful sedative, a normal sleeper who has a few drinks during a single evening will probably fall asleep faster than usual and is more likely than usual to stay asleep for the first half of the night. Before you reach for the liquor cabinet, though, you should know that the *second* half of the night can be fraught with increased awakenings and light sleep, experienced as insomnia or nonrestorative sleep. Also, the sedative effects in the first half of the night diminish after a few nights. Finally, some people are unpleasantly surprised to find that instead of sedating them, alcohol keeps them wide awake, which prevents them from falling asleep or disrupts their entire night of sleep.

Alcohol affects sleep architecture in many ways, among them reducing REM sleep during the first half of the night and in compensation increasing it during the second half. Alcohol affects sleep even when consumed hours before sleep or when the person doesn't seem to be inebriated. Most dangerous of all, using alcohol as a sleep aid can set the stage for alcoholism.

If you're in the habit of drinking alcohol before bedtime, try eliminating your drinking altogether. After a few days, your sleep may begin to improve. If you can't stop drinking all at once, try to reduce your nightly alcohol intake gradually over several weeks (use a measuring cup to control your portion). If having a drink in your hand in the evening is important for you, replace your alcoholic drink with water, decaffeinated soda, herbal tea, or fruit juice.

If you've been drinking regularly or heavily and find that you cannot reduce or stop your alcohol use, you may be suffering from alcoholism. You should consult with your primary care provider and consider enrollment in an Alcoholics Anonymous program.

Alcoholism and Sleep Problems

Alcoholism increases arousals and wakefulness during the sleep period, decreases deep sleep, and disturbs REM sleep. An alcoholic may wake in the morning feeling not only the effects of a poor night of sleep but also a hangover.

If you are an alcoholic, recovering from your problem is the most important step toward solving your sleep problems. However, sleep disturbances can persist for years after your last drink. You may experience insomnia; an EEG would show other evidence of disturbed sleep as well. More than most people, you may benefit from working with a trained sleep clinician who can give you the support and guidance you will need.

Alcohol Plus Sleep Deprivation Equal Trouble

When alcohol is combined with sleep deprivation, performance is decreased much more than it would be by either factor alone. One study showed that sleep-deprived people do as badly after three drinks as other people do after six! *Consider a person who has two drinks at a party and then drives home around midnight. Two drinks may have seemed like a safe amount of alcohol, but on this Friday night, this person is at the end of a long, hard work week and was also out late the night before. Scenarios like this cause more accidents than most people realize. Drinking and driving—always a dangerous combination—are even more deadly if you are sleep deprived.*

Alcohol and Breathing Disorders

If you have a sleep-related breathing disorder like snoring or sleep apnea, alcohol will make your condition significantly worse. Some snorers who have no signs of sleep apnea under normal conditions have sleep apnea following alcohol intake. Alcohol is a respiratory suppressant, and even a moderate amount reduces the efficiency of breathing by as much as a half. Alcohol affects breathing much more during sleep than during wakefulness. It reduces the tone of the muscles that keep the upper airway open during sleep. If you have a sleep-related breathing disorder, you should not drink alcohol.

TIP 5. STOP SMOKING

Being a nonsmoker at a gathering of smokers is like being a non-drinker at a party where everyone else is intoxicated. Because nicotine is a stimulant, the more smoking is done, the more animated and loud most conversation becomes, the more intense some reactions are, and the more hand gestures and other physical movement flail about. If you're a smoker, I bet you didn't know that, especially if you thought your smoking was helping you feel relaxed and calm.

Nicotine is a highly addictive drug. When you smoke, the nicotine in the inhaled smoke is absorbed rapidly; it reaches your brain in just seven seconds and then falls off quickly. Once you are addicted, your body lets you know, day and night, awake and asleep, that it wants another dose. The internal effects of nicotine are astonishing. Nicotine stimulates the release of norepinephrine and epinephrine, chemicals so powerful that they are used very cautiously to restart the heart after cardiac arrest. Once released in the bloodstream, these substances decrease appetite, increase heart rate, elevate blood pressure, and increase wakefulness. These effects can carry over into the sleep period. It then takes longer to fall asleep, and the number and durations of awakenings during the night increase.

If you are addicted to nicotine, your body demands regular doses. If you need a cigarette to calm down so you can sleep, or if you awaken repeatedly during the night feeling like you need a cigarette to get back to sleep, and the first thing you want in the morning is a cigarette, you are experiencing nicotine withdrawal symptoms. Smoking-waking-smoking can become an established pattern if you respond to awakenings by smoking to get back to sleep.

If you smoke and are experiencing insomnia, sleep disruption, or nonrestorative sleep, getting rid of tobacco may help significantly. Although stopping is difficult, it can be done. A lot is at stake because smoking is the source of many forms of cancer and many respiratory disorders. If you can't quit by yourself, contact your primary health provider or a local smoking-cessation program. The American Cancer Society has a list of such programs and materials that can help you, all available through the society's toll-free cancer information hotline at 1-800-ACS-2345. If you are cutting back on smoking on your own, you might begin by eliminating all smoking during the sleep period, then reducing and eliminating late-evening smoking, then early-evening smoking, then afternoon smoking, and so on. The more time you place between your last cigarette and bedtime, the better.

Nicotine patches, which help some people overcome the addiction, can sometimes disrupt sleep. The nicotine is absorbed through your skin, even while you are sleeping, and can cause arousal. Talk to your doctor about using a sixteen-hour patch, which you remove at bedtime and replace in the morning.

I have seen in my practice the dramatic difference that stopping smoking can make in the quality of sleep. For example, Donna was a middle-aged woman who smoked more than a pack of cigarettes a day. She had terrible sleep-onset and maintenance insomnia. Married to a well-to-do businessman, Donna didn't work outside the home, and she had domestic help for the household, so she had more opportunity than most to enjoy leisurely days and recreation. But Donna's sleep was so disrupted that she found it difficult to get out of bed in the morning and felt washed-out and drained all day.

When I first saw Donna, I evaluated her with a sleep log. We then initiated a smoking-cessation program with no other behavioral changes and no addition of medication. Years of sleep disruption ended when Donna's sleep returned to normal—seemingly miraculously—after just six weeks! Her last contact with me was a voice-mail message: "I hope you are having a morning as great as mine." I believe that there are many people like Donna who would experience marked improvements in sleep if they quit smoking.

TIP 6. DRINK DECAFFEINATED BEVERAGES

Caffeine is a central nervous system stimulant, a drug. In the United States, about 90 percent of caffeine comes from coffee, which contains between 50 and 150 milligrams a cup depending on how it's prepared. Anthropologists of the future may well conclude that coffee drinking was a religious ritual toward the end of the twentieth century, performed at home and in houses of worship such as Starbucks, Caribou, Dunkin' Donuts, coffee shops, and truck stops. What other beverages, besides water and a few brands of soda pop, do employers feel obligated to have on hand at all times for their employees? Then there's all the caffeine we get in tea (35 mg), cola (35–50 mg), hot cocoa (3–12 mg), and chocolate bars (5–35 mg). Beverages such as Jolt cola or Sun Bolt fruit drinks pack as much caffeine as a cup of coffee.

The reason we love caffeine so much is that it wakes us up, increases mental alertness, and quickens response time on simple motor tasks. Consumed prior to bedtime, however, caffeine can wreck havoc with sleep. Most obviously, caffeine increases the time it takes to fall asleep. How much so depends on the individual. Some people are so sensitive to caffeine that a late-afternoon or early-evening cup of coffee can leave them staring at the ceiling late into the night. In addition, caffeine increases the number of awakenings and replaces deep, delta sleep with lighter levels of sleep.

Caffeine consumption may also increase blood pressure and heart rate. These changes are most prominent when caffeine is consumed by someone who does not regularly use it, and they seem to lessen over time. However, people who use caffeine regularly may experience cardiac arrhythmia (irregular heart beats) that are a direct result of the caffeine.

Caffeine is addictive, though much less so than nicotine, so withdrawal from it can cause mood changes, dizziness, and headaches. However, these problems usually last only a few days. You may also be psychologically addicted if your coffee drinking has become ingrained in your personal, work, and social life.

If you consume caffeine and also suffer from a sleep problem, consider reducing or eliminating caffeine. You can reduce your caffeine consumption in a number of ways.

- If you normally consume caffeine in coffee or tea, switch to decaffeinated coffee or tea or a naturally caffeine-free herbal tea. These days, decaffeinated coffees are quite flavorful and difficult to distinguish from their high-test counterparts. Enlightened coffee-shop staff no longer sneer at you if you request a latte or cappuccino made with decaf coffee.
- If you feel you can't eliminate your caffeine consumption all at once, eliminate the last cup of coffee or tea that you take each day. Try this for a few weeks to see if it helps your sleep. If not, then cut back even further by eliminating midafternoon coffee, lunchtime coffee, one of your breakfast coffees, and so on.
- Another way to gradually reduce your caffeine intake is to blend caffeinated coffee and decaffeinated coffee together. You can prepare a brew that contains 75 percent caffeinated coffee and 25 percent decaffeinated coffee, and then gradually, over several weeks, reduce your caffeine percentage to 50 percent, 25 percent, and then 0.
- If you're trying to manage your caffeine intake, never trust a pot you haven't brewed yourself. Every office has its caffeine junkies who double-up the portion of coffee grounds per pot, especially

in the morning, or brew regular in the decaf pot because the regular pot was missing. Safer options are bringing decaf coffee to work with you, brewing your own in a one-cup pot at your desk, or using instant decaf.

- In a restaurant, be emphatic if you're ordering decaf, and when the coffee arrives, ask with a smile, "And you did remember to make this decaf?"
- At home, if you're trying to control the total number of cups and the timing of coffee, use a small pot that can easily be disconnected and stashed in a kitchen cabinet after your morning cup. Out of sight, out of mind!
- Watch out for caffeine in soft drinks, chocolate, and over-the-counter and prescription medications.

You may be very satisfied to exchange caffeine consumption for better sleep. However, even reformed caffeine users will occasionally fall off the wagon. When this happens, you should simply be aware of the trade-off that you may be making in your nighttime sleep and be careful to consume caffeine in moderation and as far in advance of your sleep period as possible.

TIP 7. CHECK YOUR MEDICATIONS

Many medications, both over-the-counter and prescribed, can have a profound impact on sleep. If you are taking medications and begin to have trouble with your sleep, be alert to the possibility that the sleep problem may be a side effect. Report side effects of any medications promptly to your health care provider.

Some drugs that don't affect sleep when taken alone can do so in combination with other drugs. Always let your health care provider know if you are taking over-the-counter or alternative medications in addition to prescribed medications. Drug interactions can cause serious side effects, including sleep disturbances, or make treatment less effective.

If your sleep problem is caused by a medication and is severe, your doctor may be able to change your medication, dose, or schedule. Problems with medications occur very frequently, and you aren't being a lot of trouble if you call your health provider for assistance. The magic words to say when you call are, "I am having a problem with my medication, and I think Dr. X will want to take care of this as soon as possible."

On page 48 is a list of medications that are known to affect sleep. You may find that some of the medications you are taking are listed there. In addition, new medications enter the market every week. Also, many drugs that don't cause problems alone can do so when combined with other medications. Therefore, even though the list is informative, you should always consult with your health care provider if you think your sleep problems (or other side effects) may be related to your medication.

TIP 8. LEAVE YOUR WORRIES BEHIND

When you're lying awake waiting for sleep that doesn't come, it's so tempting to begin to think. After all, the place is quiet, the phone is not likely to ring, the children are asleep, the dog doesn't want to go out, and there usually isn't any time during the day for the luxury of thinking. The problem is that *this* time is reserved for sleep. What's more, despite the elusiveness of sleep on such nights, your body, mind, and spirit are really needing sleep. They're not going to render the clear, enjoyable, productive thinking you can achieve during the day. In fact, they're going to fight back by opening Pandora's box. Look out, here they come, all those troubles that made you so tired in the first place. You'll spin your wheels mulling over what a neighbor said about the condition of your lawn or why you haven't had a date in six months. You won't solve a thing—and you will keep yourself up, maybe all night.

This pattern often occurs when going to bed is the first opportunity to think about the events of your day. Then because you're tired, it's harder to suppress disturbing thoughts.

Fortunately, techniques exist for breaking this pattern. The indigenous tribes of Central America came up with a good one long ago. They keep a set of tiny dolls, dressed in colorful scraps of fabric and each with its own identity, in a box about the size of a matchbox. At bedtime, the box is opened and the dolls taken out. Troubles and worries are whispered, one at a time, to the dolls. After every little worry has been told to the dolls, they are returned to the box and sealed in, where they will do the worrying for the person throughout the night.

A more contemporary approach is to schedule "worry time" into your daily routine. Choose any fifteen- or twenty-minute period during the day that is convenient for focusing on the thoughts or situations that seem to rise from under the bed at night. Perhaps your lunch hour, or the time during your drive to or from work, will do, but it's better to be able to sit quietly without distractions. You might identify a comfortable place in your home or on your deck or balcony where you will sit each night after dinner for twenty minutes, alone and free of distraction so that you can focus on yourself. If you think better in motion, try an evening constitutional—a short walk after dinner. Make a conscious effort to set aside your worry time each day. Anything you can do to formalize or structure this time is helpful.

If an unpleasant thought arises at bedtime or some other time during the day, acknowledge it—"This is important and I will think about it during my worry time tomorrow"—and let it go. Then, at your next scheduled worry time, make sure to focus on this thought.

If your worries awaken you during the night, tell them to go away until your next worry time. If this admonition doesn't do the trick, you might use guided imagery (explained in the next chapter) to replace worrisome thoughts with pleasant, comforting thoughts.

Another technique for dealing with worries throughout the day and night is to use a journal or notebook. Keep the journal at your bedside so that when you awaken during the night, you can jot down any concerns or disturbing thoughts you have. Just a few words or phrases can capture the essence of your concerns. Writing down the thought is a very effective way to put matters out of your mind, especially since you know that you'll have it all in writing when you sit down to your next scheduled worry time. You may also choose to use your worry time to write in the journal.

One woman kept a spiritual journal, phrasing the things that worried her as prayers or meditations. Over several years, she eventually filled several small notebooks. She found it reassuring to go back through them from time to time, writing in the margins how the things that worried her so much had been resolved and how she had grown and moved on to new challenges. She learned a lot, she said, by see-

ing that some things had never changed but had ceased to be problems because she was able to put the worry aside.

Staying Awake to Worry about Sleep

The Olympic champions of worrywarts stay awake at night to focus
exclusively on the fact that they're not asleep. These folks:

- Fear that they will not fall asleep at night
- Dread bedtime
- Focus on how they will not be able to function during the day
  without a good night's sleep
- Suspect that sleep disturbance is a sign that something is physi-
  cally or mentally wrong with them
- Spend a good bit of time each night chewing on the fact that
  repeated nights of poor sleep will affect their health or well-
  being
- Believe that one bad night will lead to many bad nights of sleep
- Are certain that normal sleepers never have a bad night's sleep

This sort of thinking seems pretty silly in the light of day (though
nearly everyone has engaged in it at some time or other). It is not
amusing, however, if it becomes a nightly occupation. If you suffer
these disruptive thoughts, you might choose to use your worry time
to revise your thinking for the better. You may also benefit from the
"cognitive retraining" technique in the next chapter. Finally, tips 9 and
10 below are especially important for you.

TIP 9. ESTABLISH A HELPFUL
PRESLEEP ROUTINE

Most people begin their day with a morning routine. Showering,
drying off, drying and styling hair, brushing teeth, shaving or putting
on makeup—they follow the same sequence day after day. Creatures
of habit, we find such routines a comforting way to ease into the day
ahead. When the routine is disrupted, we get grumpy. (Think of the
bother when a visiting relative barges into the bathroom ahead of you,
making you actually eat breakfast before you've had your shower.)

Despite how helpful and natural morning routines are, many fewer people have developed routines for closing the day. If you are having trouble falling asleep, an evening routine can really help. It is a powerful way to set the stage for sleep. Consider the possibilities. You might first have a light snack, then lay your clothes out for the next day, take a warm bath or shower, brush your teeth and comb your hair and then listen to soft or meditative music or indulge in some *light* reading (no lurid page-turner murder mysteries, no *Fun Things to Do with Calculus*). Then lights out.

The most important thing about your routine is that it begin shortly before the sleep period (at least thirty to sixty minutes before bedtime) and that it be performed in the same way every night before going to bed.

Pets are avid (sometimes militant!) supporters of routines, so you might include a few minutes getting your cat or dog settled for the night. After a few nights of this special time together, your pet will appear at the appointed hour and look woeful until you comply. If you have a family at home, everyone in the household will have a more settled, "all's well with the world" feeling if they know that when you finish your cup of herbal tea and check the doors to be sure they're locked, the day is officially over.

Avoid activities that are stimulating: completing paperwork for your job, attending to family finances, talking with a relative on the phone, or discussing important or sensitive issues with your significant other. Whatever works for you, assemble it into an orderly, comfortable, and pleasant routine (not a regimented exercise!) and designate the time when you will begin the routine each night.

Creating a ritual worked very well for Laura, a highly successful account executive with an advertising firm in Manhattan. One of the reasons for Laura's success at work was that she was willing to work late into the evening. Arriving home near midnight, she would read her mail (mostly bills), undress, and climb into bed. And then she would lay awake thinking about all of the things left undone at work, as well as things she needed to get done at home. I suggested adding a nighttime ritual. She tried it and soon reported, "It was like I was a freight train moving at top speed and then suddenly trying to stop. I had too much momentum and I couldn't end the day. Now I can gradually relax before getting into bed."

You may have the opposite problem: not enough to do during the day, followed by a sedentary evening. This pattern may obscure the transition between what you expect your body to do in the evening and what you expect it to do during the sleep period. If the evening is too quiet, you may find that as you watch TV, listen to music, or read, you are dozing off, and then you have to wake up so you can go to bed. This routine is not helpful, especially if you have difficulty sleeping once you get to bed.

Ideally, you should sustain your daytime activity until you are ready to begin your presleep routine and then complete the routine before getting into bed. Napping or dozing off in the evening is as ruinous to your sleep as having a sandwich right before supper would be to your appetite. If you have this problem, try engaging in some activity during the time that you usually doze off. Instead of watching TV, go for a walk or play a game with a family member.

TIP 10. DON'T TRY TOO HARD

Some people who have trouble sleeping take the "drill sergeant approach": It is time to sleep, and by gum, I am going to stay in this bed and *sleep!* This approach is counterproductive because it puts your mind and body on alert. The harder you try, the more awake you will become. What's worse, this approach can foster troubling thoughts ("What's wrong with me?") and nurture insomnia.

So relax. And stop staring at the clock. Watching the clock helps the problem, not you. Avoid all time cues between the time that you get into bed at night and the time that you arise in the morning. Store your wristwatch in a drawer, turn all the clocks away from you or cover them with a scarf, and stop all chiming clocks from chiming during your sleep period. There really is no need for you to be aware of time while you are sleeping.

Use your own impression of your nighttime sleep to assess whether it has been a good or bad night. Better yet, use a sleep log. (But as always, use estimates, not the clock, to gauge the times.)

* 6 *

Behavioral Treatments
for Insomnia

If you have insomnia, your first steps should be to keep a sleep log, establish your bedtime and rise time, and apply the ten tips for better sleep. If your sleep problems still persist, the next step is one or more techniques that can change your sleep behaviors. This chapter explains a variety of options, ranging from simple to demanding. You can use these therapies on your own or with the help of a sleep clinic or psychologist. The techniques are

- Stimulus control therapy
- Sleep restriction therapy
- Relaxation therapies
- Cognitive therapy

All of these therapies are known to be effective in the treatment of insomnia. *They work best when applied in the context of a regular sleep period and good sleep habits, so I advise that you use them after you have established a regular bedtime and rise time and in conjunction with the ten tips of better sleep.*
When you apply a behavioral technique, your sleep may not improve substantially for four to six weeks. Some people report changes occurring much earlier, and a few people don't experience improve-

ment for more than six weeks. How well you respond depends upon the nature of your insomnia, the treatment techniques that you try and, most of all, your persistence in following through. Since it takes time to see consistent improvement when you're using these treatments, many people become frustrated and discontinue the treatment before realizing any benefit. They then conclude that "this treatment just doesn't work for me" and are very unlikely to try it again.

Continue to keep a sleep log while you're trying behavioral methods. The log will show clearly any improvement. You should keep one sleep log or diary before starting treatment, one covering several weeks while you modify your sleep time or sleep habits, and one covering several weeks of behavioral treatment.

STIMULUS CONTROL THERAPY

As we discussed earlier, many people with insomnia spend too much time awake in bed, lying awake for long periods while working at falling asleep, staying in bed during awakenings during the sleep period, or engaging in other activities in bed. All of these responses to insomnia condition your body to respond to the bed and sleep environment by becoming wide awake.

The first psychological experiments in classical conditioning were done by Ivan Pavlov, a Russian scientist and Nobel prize winner. Pavlov noticed that when he presented a dog with a piece of meat, the dog salivated. In his most famous experiment, he rang a bell every time he gave the dog meat. After several pairings, Pavlov had only to ring the bell to prompt the dog to salivate.

No, we are not going to use a bell to help you sleep, but Pavlov's model of conditioning explains why using your bed for anything other than sleep can promote insomnia. If your bed or sleep environment is paired with wakefulness or some other activity, you will begin to associate the bed with wakefulness or the activity. When you get into bed, instead of feeling comfortable and relaxed, you will become wide awake.

Dr. Richard Bootzin, currently a professor at the University of Arizona, had a theory that *reducing* time awake in bed could reduce this harmful association. He developed stimulus control therapy, which has been used for several years with remarkable success in treating insomnia. The instructions are simple. I've modified them slightly for your use.

1. Avoid your bed, and preferably your bedroom, for anything other than sleep or sexual activity.
2. Get into bed at your predetermined bedtime, or later if you're not sleepy at your usual bedtime. (If you have insomnia, it's better to spend less time in bed than to lie awake.)
3. Allow yourself ten to fifteen minutes to fall asleep. Estimate this time. Don't use a clock or other time cue.
4. If you're not asleep within ten to fifteen minutes, get out of bed, go to another room, and engage in a quiet activity until you think you might be able to sleep.
5. Return to bed. Then repeat steps two through four. Repeat this procedure as often as necessary throughout the night.
6. Get out of bed in the morning at your predetermined rise time. If you're awake before your rise time, you can get out of bed and start your day. Don't allow yourself to sleep beyond your predetermined rise time.
7. Do not nap during the day.

As you can see, you're allowed to remain awake in bed only for a short time before falling asleep. If you wake for more than a few minutes during the night, you have to get out of bed until you feel sleepy. This procedure helps to break the learned association between being awake and being in bed. As a result, it helps to break the ongoing pattern of insomnia.

You may find that you have a difficult time with this procedure at first. If you're like most people, you're likely to get out of bed several times a night for the first several nights of treatment. *Your sleep will generally improve as time goes on;* keep this in mind during the early weeks, when it may be difficult to tell if the program is really working.

Be prepared to deal with daytime sleepiness. In the beginning, because the treatment will result in extended periods of wakefulness *out of bed* during the night, you may get even less sleep than usual. Actually, the daytime sleepiness is a positive development because it will promote sleep the next night. After one or two nights of getting less sleep, you are likely to rebound and get more sleep on the following night. However, be very careful to avoid any hazardous activity if you're sleepy during the day. Make sure that your sleepiness doesn't put others at risk; be particularly careful not to drive while you are fatigued and sleepy.

At first, the daytime fatigue and sleepiness may affect your ability to function at home and at work. It's a good idea to let those at home know what you (and they) are in for. And while you're at it, enlist some help. While you're using this therapy, you sometimes won't want to get out of bed when you're supposed to or will want to return to bed early or sleep late. Just about everyone struggles with this urge, but you will have the greatest chance of success if you follow the rules.

If you've tried stimulus control therapy before without success, it's worth another try. This time, be sure to follow all of the rules, all of the time.

SLEEP RESTRICTION THERAPY

Sleep restriction therapy is another very successful behavioral treatment for insomnia. Like stimulus control therapy, sleep restriction therapy requires that you limit your time in bed. However, the philosophy behind sleep restriction therapy is different. There's no supposition that conditioning plays a role in insomnia. Sleep restriction therapy is based on the observation that people with insomnia simply spend too much time in bed. According to Dr. Arthur J. Spielman, people with insomnia can have shallow sleep that is spread out over too great a time period. If you recall our discussion of sleep architecture, sleep without depth is neither healthful nor restorative.

Think of sleep as water in a swimming pool. If a pool measuring 10 feet by 10 feet and 8 feet deep is filled with water, it will be deep enough for safe diving. However, if a pool measuring 100 feet by 100 feet by 8 feet deep is filled with the same amount of water, you'll want to remove the diving board before inviting any friends who are lawyers over for a swim. The goal of sleep restriction therapy is to make deeper sleep possible by shrinking the dimensions of your "sleeping pool."

The first step in sleep restriction therapy is to keep a sleep log for seven to ten days. Calculate your average time in bed and your average total sleep time. (If you need a refresher course on these calculations, turn back to chapter 4.) Let's look at how sleep restriction therapy worked out for Martina, a real estate agent who had had a long struggle with insomnia.

Martina was trying to get to bed at a fairly regular time, around

MARTINA'S SLEEP LOG

Date	Bedtime	Time until sleep onset	Awakenings (number, total length)	Wake time	Rise time	Naps yesterday (number, total length)	Total time in bed	Total time asleep
5/1	10:30 P.M.	1h	0	7:30 A.M.	7:30 A.M.	0	9	8
5/2	10:45 P.M.	45m	0	7:30 A.M.	7:45 A.M.	0	9	8
5/3	11:30 P.M.	1h:30m	0	8:00 A.M.	8:00 A.M.	0	8.5	7
5/4	10:30 P.M.	2h	0	7:30 A.M.	7:30 A.M.	0	9	7
5/5	8:30 P.M.	0m	1 (1h)	9:30 A.M.	9:30 A.M.	0	13	12
5/6	10:30 P.M.	30m	1 (30m)	7:30 A.M.	7:30 A.M.	0	9	8
5/7	10:30 P.M.	2h:30m	0	5:30 A.M.	7:30 A.M.	0	9	4.5
5/8	10:30 P.M.	45m	0	6:45 A.M.	7:30 A.M.	0	9	7.5
5/9	10:30 P.M.	1h:15m	0	6:00 A.M.	7:30 A.M.	0	9	6.25
5/10	12:30 A.M.	0	0	7:00 A.M.	7:30 A.M.	0	7	6.5

10:30 but was having a lot of difficulty getting to sleep and staying asleep. She did manage to get up consistently at 7:30 A.M. except on the fifth day, when exhaustion overtook her and she overslept until 9:30 A.M.—arriving, to her great embarrassment, an hour late for a client's closing and looking every bit as tired as she was. The sleep log revealed the following:

- Martina's average bedtime was 10:37 P.M.
- Her average rise time was 7:46 A.M.
- Her average total time in bed was 9 hours and 9 minutes (549 minutes).
- Her average time asleep was 7 hours and 29 minutes (449 minutes).

Martina believed that she had to get up by at least 7:30 A.M. to meet the demands of her clients. She thought she probably should be getting up even earlier on the weekends, which are exceptionally busy in real estate. Because Martina did occasionally oversleep and she felt fatigued during the day, she thought she needed more sleep than her insomnia was permitting her to get.

Since her actual average time in bed was 9 hours and 9 minutes and her average sleep time was 7 hours and 29 minutes, she was awake in bed an average of 1 hour and 40 minutes a night. We began correcting Martina's sleep problem by reducing her average total nightly time in bed to her current average sleep time, 7 hours and 29 minutes.

It was best for Martina to trim her time in bed by going to bed later. Her new bedtime was based on her predetermined rise time. Counting backwards from 7:30 A.M., we found that Martina's ideal bedtime was about midnight. However, she felt that going to bed at midnight would result in wasted time in the evening, since she didn't have any meaningful activities after 10:30 P.M. So she decided to go to bed at 11:00 P.M. and rise at 6:30 A.M., which gave her an extra hour in the morning to think and prepare for her day. She was then at the starting gate for the rest of the sleep restriction therapy program. Here are the instructions:

1. Subtract your average total nightly sleep time from your average total nightly time in bed. This indicates the excessive amount of time that you are spending in bed.
2. Eliminate the excess time you spend in bed. In our example, Martina should be in bed for a total of approximately 7.5 hours. This is not necessarily a permanent change in her schedule. She may find that 7.5 hours is too long or too short. It's best to trim hours off your bedtime by going to bed later.
3. You can always go to bed later than your prescribed bedtime, but never earlier. You can always rise earlier than your prescribed bedtime, but never later.
4. Do not nap during the day.
5. Keep a sleep log for seven to ten days. Then calculate your new average total nightly time in bed and your average total nightly sleep time.

6. Calculate your sleep efficiency by dividing total average time in bed by total average time asleep (use minutes). Sleep efficiency is the percentage of time spent asleep in bed. If your sleep efficiency reaches 85 percent, the treatment is working effectively.

7. If your sleep efficiency is less than 85 percent, reduce your time in bed once again, this time by the amount of time your sleep log says you're now spending awake in bed. For example, one person came to our center for help because he was spending 8 hours in bed, but sleeping only 6. After reducing his time in bed by the wakeful 2 hours, he then was spending 6 hours in bed—but sleeping 5. As the next step, we reduced his time in bed by 1 more hour. He then was spending 5 hours in bed each night. He kept a sleep log for another 7 days. He reported excitedly that he was falling asleep right away and staying asleep all night.

8. This process may be repeated as often as necessary. However, it's not advisable to reduce your average total nightly time in bed to less than 4 hours.

Before embarking on sleep restriction, Martina's sleep efficiency was 82 percent (449 minutes divided by 549 minutes). This was too low, so Martina had to reduce her time in bed by 1 hour and 40 minutes, the time she was spending awake during the sleep period. She kept a sleep log for another seven to ten days and then computed her new sleep efficiency. In Martina's case, her sleep efficiency improved to more than 90 percent! Though Martina had to reduce her time in bed to achieve these results, having to make such a drastic reduction is rare. Be forewarned, while sleep restriction is a simple procedure, implementing it can be very difficult. It is considered successful if you achieve a single, consolidated episode of sleep during the night, even if it's a shorter episode than desired. Even so, most people who go through sleep restriction therapy are quite happy—as Martina was—to spend less time tossing and turning and watching the hours pass by.

Once you have achieved a sleep efficiency of 85 percent or better and have sustained this efficiency for a few weeks, you can begin to extend your total nightly sleep time. This is done by increasing your average total nightly time in bed in fifteen-minute increments. Try increasing your time in bed and then carefully evaluate your response.

If you fill that extra time with sleep, you may attempt another increase. However, when your sleep efficiency falls below 85 percent, stop making increases. At this point, you've probably gained the maximum benefit from sleep restriction therapy.

During the early days, when sleep restriction is most frustrating, enlist the support and encouragement of a family member or friend. Keep in mind that the difficulties you experience early will give way to more consolidated, deeper, and longer sleep episodes later if you continue with the treatment.

* ✸ ☾ ✸ ☾ ✸ ☾ ✸ ☾ ✸ ☾ ✸ ☾ ✸ ☾ ✸

Combined Stimulus Control Therapy and Sleep Restriction Therapy

Sometimes it helps to combine the principles of both stimulus control therapy and sleep restriction therapy. Avoid combining therapies until you have at least four to six weeks of experience with one of them. *Start by trying either stimulus control or sleep restriction therapy. Each treatment is usually challenging, difficult, and effective all by itself. Burdening yourself with too many demands can cause you to abandon the method or can lead to poor results. However, a combination may work in one of the following cases.*

- *If you began by using the stimulus control procedure and find that you have been repeatedly getting out of bed even after several weeks of treatment, you may be allowing yourself altogether too much time in bed. This is an appropriate time to apply sleep restriction principles. You can reduce your average total nightly time in bed to maximize the result that you'll get from the stimulus control procedure.*
- *On the other hand, if you began by using the sleep restriction therapy and find that you have been awakening frequently during your allowed sleep period, you may wish to apply stimulus control principles. Instead of lying awake in bed during your prescribed sleep period, you can lie awake for only ten to fifteen minutes and then get out of bed according to the stimulus control procedure. This technique can give you the added boost that you need to maximize the effectiveness of your treatment.*

RELAXATION THERAPIES

Many kinds of relaxation therapies have helped people with insomnia. Relaxation therapies improve sleep by reducing mental or physical tension.

Some research has shown that people with high levels of muscle tension respond better to relaxation techniques than other people do. However, these results are not definite, and many sleep specialists believe that relaxation techniques help even those without muscle tension. The techniques provide comfort and can be quite soothing even if your insomnia is due to a medical or psychological disorder or another cause. These techniques have been effective for many people and are considered valuable additions to behavioral treatment programs.

Many of us have never learned, or have lost the ability, to relax. We move from one activity to the next, slowing down only a few moments before getting into bed at night. Losing the ability to relax fully just prior to sleep onset, or during awakenings from sleep, can profoundly affect the quality of your sleep. Tension can make it more difficult to improve your sleep even if you follow carefully the instructions for sleep scheduling, good sleep habits, and the behavioral treatments for insomnia. Therefore, adding relaxation skills to your repertoire can improve your overall response to sleep treatment. The point of practicing relaxation techniques during the day is that you will learn how to re-create those feelings when you get into bed at night.

Relaxation therapies include simple relaxation, meditation, yoga, abdominal breathing, progressive muscle relaxation, biofeedback, and other approaches. It's difficult to predict which would work best for you because responses are so individual. Read through them and see which ones appeal most to you. Do you like technology? If so, biofeedback might be just the thing. Are you drawn to Eastern philosophy? Yoga or tai chi might work well. And so on.

Start with one of the simpler techniques rather than one that takes a considerable amount of time and practice.If simple relaxation procedures don't provide the level of relaxation you desire or don't improve your sleep, you may want to try the more advanced procedures.

Quiet Time

If you believe that you have the ability to relax but rarely allow your-self the time to do so, you may simply need to schedule a quiet time during the day reserved exclusively for relaxation. Select a comfort-able place where you can sit or recline. Avoid all possibilities of in-terruption so that this relaxation time is your own. Let your family know that you don't wish to be disturbed, unplug the phone, and do anything else that will ensure your solitude. Take advantage of your quiet time for twenty to thirty minutes each day.

Once you have selected the place for your quiet time, set the stage for relaxation. Whenever possible, dress in loose, comfortable cloth-ing, play some soft music, burn some incense, or open a window to take advantage of a slight breeze. What you do to create a relaxing mood is up to you, but it's important to think about what you find relaxing. You can sit or recline during your quiet time, but avoid lying down. Quiet time should not be used for dozing or napping.

Many people wonder if watching television, reading, or engaging in some other quiet activity is advisable during quiet time. I recom-mend against such activities. During quiet time you want to free your-self from all potential distractions and focus on the pleasant sensation of relaxation. External stimulation tends to take away this focus. How-ever, you can certainly enhance your relaxation with pleasant, com-forting thoughts or guided imagery (see below).

If you have young children at home, you might reserve their nap time as your quiet time, instead of running another load of laundry and mopping the kitchen floor. If you're a student, you can take your quiet time in the library. Just put down your pencil and focus on your-self. If you work outside the home, you might be able to schedule a getaway during your lunchtime. Have a quick sandwich and then in-dulge in your quiet time in a local library, park, or garden. If you work close to home, you might take your quiet time in your favorite chair at home after a quick lunch.

After you've learned to relax during the day, you can carry over your lessons to the night, helping yourself relax before getting into bed at night and during nighttime awakenings.

Meditation

For centuries, people have used the purposeful contemplation called meditation to achieve relaxation and find inner tranquillity. There are several different forms of meditation, but all of them are directed at gaining mastery over one's thoughts. Some schools of meditation employ a mantra, breathing exercise, or special position.

If you have never tried meditation but would like to experience it, here are a couple of techniques to try. One technique is to try to keep your mind blank. You can imagine a dark space without anything in it, or perhaps even a blank wall. Keep your mind free of all thoughts. Intrusive thoughts must be forced out of your internal blank space.

Another technique is to allow thoughts to enter your mind, but don't linger on any one thought for too long. Let your mind wander without direction and follow your thoughts in whatever direction they take you. This exercise is a mental version of browsing in a library. Many thoughts appear and disappear as you move slowly through your interior space. The thoughts that give you pause are looked at more closely. The ones that don't appeal to you are replaced "on the shelf." The appealing ones should be "read"—i.e., focused on more fully.

If you want to explore meditation further, you can do so through books or through group or private lessons from a practitioner.

Yoga and Tai Chi

Yoga has enjoyed popularity as an enriching and relaxing experience for centuries. Yoga facilitates relaxation with particular body positions. Some yoga postures, like the lotus position, are easily assumed. Others require muscle stretching and flexibility.

Tai chi is an ancient Chinese discipline. A daily ritual of gentle movement is joined with meditation to achieve spiritual peace and physical relaxation. Tai chi is learned by working with a master, individually, or in a class.

Stretching Exercises

If Eastern philosophies aren't your cup of tea, you can also get the benefits of physical relaxation by doing some simple stretching exercises. Gently stretch your muscles and then completely relax them.

Here are some examples of exercises that can be done during the day with the intent that their benefits will be carried over into the night. You can also do stretching exercises just before going to bed. The exercises should be done gently and slowly. Overworking and stressing your muscles may worsen, rather than improve, sleep. These exercises are not intended to be an aerobic workout. Some can be done at your desk or at other moments snatched during the day. Breathe slowly in and out as you do them.

- **Roll.** Roll your head and neck in a circular motion. Rotate your hips, hands, and feet. Roll each for a couple of minutes and then allow the muscle to relax.
- **Stretch.** 1. Clasp your hands in front of you with your fingers intertwined and your palms out. Stretch your arms in front of you and then raise them over your head. Do this exercise slowly and then let your muscles rest and relax. 2. Hold your arms straight out at your sides. Bend over as if you are going to touch your toes—how far you reach is not important. Dangle your arms like strands of cooked spaghetti. Move your arms around a bit and allow them to feel heavy. When you resume an upright position you will feel that your neck and shoulders, back, and arms have all stretched slightly. 3. Lie on your back. Bring your knees up to your chest. Hold this position for a few seconds and then release. Notice the slight stretch in your legs and buttocks.
- **Press.** While lying on the floor with your arms at your side, your knees bent, and your feet flat on the floor, you can do several simple isometric exercises. 1. Press your head backward against the floor, stretching the muscles of your head and neck. 2. Press the palms of your hands against the floor, stretching the muscles of your arms and shoulders. 3. Press the soles of your feet downward against the floor, stretching your thighs and calves. Tense each muscle for a few seconds and then allow it to relax. Repeat the tension and release several times during each relaxation exercise session for the maximum benefit.

If you want to explore stretching further, you can learn more exercises through books or through a class at a health club or recreation center.

Massage

If you've ever had a massage, you know how truly relaxing it can be. A massage is especially helpful if your muscles are tense. If you spring for a professional massage, be sure to tell the masseuse if you have any injury, arthritis, fibromyalgia, or other musculoskeletal condition.

If you're having trouble falling asleep, you can ask your spouse or bed partner to help you by giving you a ten-minute massage. Ask that you be massaged from head to toe, including your head, neck, shoulders, back, arms, and legs. Tell the person what feels good to you. A massage doesn't have to be performed by a brute. A gentle massage can be just as relaxing as one performed by someone with strong hands. Since massage is a relaxing prelude to sleep, it's fine to have your massage in bed just before turning the lights out.

If you don't have someone to help you, you can still get a good massage from someone who knows you very well—yourself! With the fingers of both hands, make a small, circular motion across your scalp, forehand, face, and then along the base of your neck and shoulders. A personal vibrator, available from your pharmacy or a department store, can help you reach muscles, such as your back, that you could not comfortably reach otherwise.

The Quieting Response

Several years ago, Dr. Charles Stroebel developed a technique that he called the quieting response that combines mental imagery and body movement to achieve relaxation. The quieting response can be used during the day to help promote relaxation and can also be used at night while lying in bed just prior to lights out. *When using this technique for insomnia, your best results will be obtained if you have daytime practice sessions in addition to using the procedure at night.*

Here are the instructions for the quieting response.

1. Sit or lie in a comfortable position with your eyes closed.
2. Breathe quietly, easily, and deeply for thirty to forty seconds.
3. Lift your arms slowly above your head and breathe deeply. Lower your arms to your sides and breathe out, going completely limp. Then hold your arms as if praying. Take a deep breath and press your hands together until they tremble. Breathe out and go com-

pletely limp. Take the prayer position with your hands about three inches apart. Notice the flow of warmth between your hands. Take a deep breath, bring your arms to your sides, and relax.

4. Imagine sunlight on top of your head.
5. Imagine your body as an empty bottle.
6. Let the warm sunlight slowly fill this bottle, beginning with your toes and feet. Fill your legs, abdomen, and so on.
7. When heavy warmth reaches your shoulders, let it flow into your arms, hands, and fingers.
8. Notice your breathing—slow, regular, easy, calm.
9. With your eyes still closed, focus just beyond the tip of your nose. Let the sunlight on your head change to the misty light of a winter moon. Repeat this phrase: Cool, alert mind; warm, heavy body.

Like other techniques, the quieting response works best if you practice, practice, practice. For more information on this technique, see Dr. Stroebel's book *Quieting Reflex Training for Adults.*

Abdominal Breathing

Another relaxation technique is abdominal breathing—deep, rhythmic breathing that completely fills the lungs. Many of us normally take short, shallow breaths that don't fill our lungs fully. Abdominal breathing can make you feel calm and comfortable and can physically relax your body by reducing muscle tension and lowering heart rate.

Deep, rhythmic breathing can help you to fall asleep a bit faster and may shorten the duration of nighttime awakenings. You should practice the technique a few times before using it for insomnia. It is simple and can be practiced just about anywhere. You can learn it quite well by practicing for just a few minutes, twice a day, for several days in a row.

1. At first, practice this breathing technique lying down. Make sure that the clothing that you're wearing doesn't restrict the movement of your abdominal muscles. Place your feet slightly apart.
2. Start breathing regularly through your nose with your mouth closed. Then begin to focus on your abdominal muscles. Stretch your diaphragm to slowly draw in a breath. You should see your stomach begin to rise. Draw the breath in gradually, as if you're trying to fill your lungs from the very bottom all the way up to the top.

3. Once your lungs are full, hold the breath for one second and then gradually exhale through your nose to the count of four. Repeat this procedure at a rate that you find comfortable.

You may have trouble at first knowing whether you're actually using your diaphragm. Also, many people expand their chests when breathing, rather than breathing deep down. Place one hand gently over your abdomen and another on your chest. Then while practicing the technique, watch and feel your hands. The one on your abdomen should move as you breathe, and the one on your chest should remain stable. Once you get the hang of it, abdominal breathing is an easy relaxation technique and is remarkably effective.

Progressive Muscle Relaxation

Progressive muscle relaxation is a sequence of tensing and then completely relaxing groups of muscles. First developed as a treatment for anxiety and hyperarousal, it has also helped some people with insomnia. Though there is enough evidence indicating that it is a useful technique, no one knows exactly why progressive muscle relaxation works. It may work best for people who have high amounts of muscle tension to start with.

Mastering progressive muscle relaxation takes ten to twelve weeks and considerable diligence. For several weeks, you have to practice one or two times a day. When people fail, it's usually because they are unable to adhere to the schedule of regular practice. One way to encourage yourself to practice regularly is to set aside a specific time each day, as if you were scheduling a doctor's appointment. For the first practice session, you'll need forty-five to sixty minutes, but later, you will need only about fifteen minutes. On the positive side, your practice sessions will be pleasant, comforting, and most of all, relaxing. Like other forms of relaxation therapy, progressive muscle relaxation training should be done in a quiet, comfortable place free of noise and distractions.

Progressive muscle relaxation therapy involves identifying various muscle groups in your body and then tensing and relaxing each group in a specific order. A typical sequence is dominant hand and forearm; other hand and forearm; dominant biceps and triceps; other biceps and triceps; forehead, upper cheeks, and nose; lower cheeks and jaw;

neck and throat; chest/shoulders/upper back; abdomen; dominant thigh; other thigh; dominant calf; other calf; dominant foot; other foot. When you tense the muscles, they should feel hard and a bit uncomfortable. After five or so seconds, you abruptly release the tension and feel the muscles loosen, unwind, smooth out, and relax. During the relaxation phase, you should feel placid, calm, and tranquil.

As you master the technique, you can combine the muscles into progressively larger groups. At the highest level, a "countdown" will bring on the relaxation response without having to tense and relax any muscle groups at all.

If you are interested in this therapy, you can learn it from a behavioral therapist, usually a psychologist.

Once your relaxation skills are well developed, you can use them to improve your sleep, particularly for wakefulness during the night. However, if your skills are not good and you start using them while you lie awake in bed at night, insomnia may overpower your abilities. You may get frustrated and think the techniques can't help you, when actually they can. Be sure to learn the relaxation technique well before taking it to bed with you, and if you choose to have a second practice session during the day, don't do it while lying in bed just before going to sleep.

Biofeedback

Biofeedback is a relaxation technique that teaches you to gauge and alter various physical states of your body. You learn it by being hooked up to a machine that sends back a constant flow of visual or sound signals about your muscle activity, body temperature, skin resistance, or other aspect of your body. You apply your mental processes to try to alter a specific state and then get immediate feedback on whether you have been successful. For example, by receiving continuous signals about the tension in a particular muscle, your mind can learn how to raise or lower your muscle activity and control the tension.

This alternative medical treatment has moved into the mainstream and is often recommended by doctors as a treatment for several disorders. Feedback on muscle tension has been used to treat anxiety, tension headache, chronic pain, movement disorders, communication disorders, and incontinence. Biofeedback on body temperature can treat migraine headache and Raynaud's disease. Other forms of biofeedback, such as heart rate and blood pressure biofeedback, are sometimes used to treat cardiovascular disorders, including high blood pressure and irregular heartbeat.

Most important to our purposes, biofeedback therapy has been successfully used to treat insomnia. It has shortened the time to sleep onset and improved sleep continuity. The treatment may work best for people who hold tension in their muscles.

Biofeedback is accomplished with the aid of a trained therapist and sophisticated equipment. Today most biofeedback therapists use a computer that monitors several physical states at one time and provides audio feedback through a speaker or video feedback on a screen. Your therapist will help you control and shape your responses to the information that you're gaining through biofeedback.

Many people find the guidance of the therapist invaluable, but if you would rather work alone, you have the option of purchasing biofeedback equipment. Small, inexpensive biofeedback units can perform the same basic functions as the computerized systems in the therapist's office. Some of these systems come with instructions and workbooks to help you develop your own home-treatment program. To get the best of both worlds, use a home unit to practice the biofeedback training you have done with a therapist.

If you decide to pursue biofeedback therapy, it's important to consider the role it should occupy in your treatment. Most people with insomnia should try more basic treatments first. You should maintain a sleep log, follow the ten tips for good sleep habits, pursue a course of stimulus control therapy or sleep restriction therapy, and use simple relaxation procedures. Only after these steps have been taken should you introduce more aggressive relaxation techniques such as progressive muscle relaxation therapy or biofeedback therapy. Also, consider whether or not you think psychological or physical tension is underlying your insomnia. If so, biofeedback therapy is more likely to help you.

If you decide to try biofeedback therapy, you'll probably follow a structured course of treatment. During your first session, you'll be connected to the biofeedback apparatus for a baseline reading of your physical data. During the course of biofeedback treatment you'll be able to gauge your progress against these starting figures.

Once baseline data has been gathered, you'll become familiar with

the biofeedback apparatus by listening to the auditory feedback (usually a tone) or watching the video monitor. Instead of trying to relax
immediately, get a feel for the biofeedback system by simply monitoring the signals. For example, what makes the tone go up? What
makes it go down? What happens when you have a pleasant thought?
A disturbing thought? What happens when you tense your muscle?
What happens when you allow them to rest?

Once you have become familiar with the equipment and your
physical responses, you can proceed with the biofeedback therapy.
You will begin with the muscles of your forearm, which many people
find easiest to regulate. Electrodes are placed over the muscles of the
forearm and then connected to the biofeedback unit. You'll focus on
relaxing the muscles while listening to a tone or watching a video
monitor. Your objective will be to lower the tone or to cause the
image on the video monitor to change (usually a line graph that you
want to drop to a lower level). You'll probably employ visual images,
statements to yourself, or special breathing techniques.

After you've learned to relax your forearm, you'll probably move
on to the forehead. Mastering this skill will probably take several sessions. You will decrease the tension in these muscles to progressively
lower levels. Once you've learned these exercises well, you and your
therapist may identify other muscles that seem tense and begin work
on those areas.

If muscle biofeedback doesn't provide the result that you desire,
you can go further to thermal or electrodermal biofeedback. In thermal
feedback, a sensor on a fingertip communicates temperature changes
to the biofeedback unit. You learn to increase your hand temperature
by increasing the flow of blood to the area. Electrodermal biofeedback also uses a fingertip sensor, this time to measure changes in your
skin's electrical conductance (no shocks are involved). The sensor is
very sensitive to changes in sweat gland activity and can detect tension and anxiety. Your objective is to achieve the lowest possible
electrodermal response. Achieving success with thermal or electrodermal biofeedback can take several sessions. However, the ability to
control these variables often means that you've reached a deep level
of relaxation.

Successful biofeedback usually takes regular, weekly appointments
with a therapist. The key to both short-term and long-term success

is to practice the relaxation technique between sessions (with or without a home biofeedback unit). You must learn the skill well before you attempt to use it to combat your insomnia. If you try to use it before you master the skill, you may find yourself frustrated and eager to abandon the treatment.

Guided Imagery

Guided imagery, which promotes relaxation through mental images, can be used alone or in conjunction with other relaxation techniques. You choose a scene that is relaxing to you and picture yourself there in great detail. You might imagine yourself lying on an ocean beach on a hot summer's day, lying among the tall grass and flowers in a lush meadow, or enjoying the sensation of a cool rain or the first snowfall. Perhaps you'd like to relive a scene from your childhood. One of my patients had fond memories of long bus rides with his father, so would imagine all of the elements of a bus ride. He could recall the clinking of the coins going through the slot, the feel of the cracked leather seats, the rumble of the bus as it rode down the streets, and the sights and sounds of the town.

To try guided imagery, select a scene that is meaningful to you. Sit or lie back, close your eyes, and then begin developing that scene in your mind. Imagine every last detail. Let's say that you would like to imagine yourself lying on a beach. Instead of holding a static picture in your mind, try to bring the scene to life. Feel the pressure of your back, hind quarters, and legs on the towel that you carefully placed on the sand. Notice the warmth of the sun on your skin, the cool breeze, the smell of the salty air, the distant sounds of children playing and seagulls calling. Feel the grains of sand on your hands and feet, the movement of your hair as it's blown by the wind and sand. Experience the taste in your mouth, the sound of your own heartbeat, the rhythm of your own breathing. Keep on developing this scene further and further, until you can go no more. You should be able to occupy yourself for fifteen or twenty minutes with such pleasant images.

If your mind starts to wander, don't be alarmed. Losing your attention is especially likely when you're a beginner. Try focusing a little harder on the details of your pleasant scene. If that doesn't help, choose a different scene. If you use guided imagery regularly, develop several scenes rather than using the same one each time. If you're having trouble coming up with more than one or two scenes, get some help from a magazine. Find photographs of distant places that you might enjoy or appealing vacation spots. Use those photographs as the foundation for your next guided imagery session.

Guided imagery using scenes from the outer world can help you relax in general, which can help with insomnia. You can replace worries and musings that are keeping you awake with pleasant trips to relaxing places.

You can also use guided imagery in a more direct way by visualizing that you are free from insomnia. You can imagine that you are taking a trip inside your own brain to the place that promotes wakefulness and sleep. Picture yourself slowing down the cellular activity and allowing yourself to be consumed by the overwhelming power of the areas that promote sleep. If you are using a sleeping medication, you can imagine it finding its way to the appropriate areas. Envision yourself free of the burdens of insomnia.

COGNITIVE THERAPY

Cognitive therapists treat insomnia by replacing harmful thoughts and beliefs about sleep (which they call maladaptive cognitions) with more positive, realistic thoughts. Cognitive therapy helps people evaluate their beliefs about insomnia, its causes, and its effects. If you are interested in this approach to insomnia, you can work with a psychologist or sleep specialist trained in this technique. Another approach is to read the book *Insomnia: Psychological Assessment and Management* by Dr. Charles Morin of the Universite Laval in Quebec, Canada.

Here are some examples of harmful thoughts and more useful replacements:

Harmful thought: I think my sleep is poor because I'm getting older.
Underlying belief: Problems falling asleep and staying asleep go hand in hand with aging.
Adaptive, realistic thought: Aging can change your sleep, but you need not sleep poorly, and insomnia is not inevitable.

Harmful thought: I've lost control over my sleep and I must resume control at once.
Underlying belief: You can't sleep unless you are in control.
Adaptive, realistic thought: Sleep is a biological process that will express itself under the right conditions. Don't try to force sleep to come. It will come if you set the stage for it, such as by following the ten tips for a good night.

Do you have some "maladaptive cognitions" of your own? If so, write them down along with the underlying beliefs that may support them. Then refer to this book or other sources to gain the information that you require to derive adaptive and realistic thoughts about your sleep. This process may seem simplistic, but you'll be surprised how much it can help you deal with insomnia.

* 7 *

Using Sleeping Pills Wisely

Medications can be an effective treatment for insomnia and other sleep problems, especially when used as part of an overall sleep program. Though not a magical fix for sleep problems, they may be able to help you resolve your sleep problems. If you have insomnia, you should decide whether medications might help you. You may have to weigh the pros and cons and consider carefully any reservations you've had in the past. This chapter will help you make intelligent choices and develop effective strategies for using sleeping pills to treat insomnia.

ABOUT SLEEPING PILLS

A *sleeping pill* is any medication that is used to promote sleep, usually to treat insomnia. A wide range of sleeping pills are available today, but they all belong to just a few drug classes:

- Barbiturates, sedating prescription drugs that depress the central nervous system and respiration, affect the heart rate, and decrease blood pressure and temperature. They are never prescribed to new users today, and some older people who still take them might benefit from switching to another medication.

- Benzodiazepines, sedative/hypnotic drugs (*hypnotic* simply means they induce sleep).
- Non-benzodiazepine hypnotics, drugs that are not members of the benzodiazepine class, but are used to promote sleep.
- Sedating antidepressants, used both to relieve depression and in low doses as sleep aids.
- Over-the-counter sleep aids, usually antihistamines.
- "Natural" sleep aids, such as melatonin and herbs.

Later, you'll learn more about these various options, but the key point for now is that more than one kind of sleeping pill is available. Drugs vary widely in effectiveness, side effects, adverse effects, and overall safety—both within each group and among the groups. Consequently, many people—including health professionals—are sometimes confused about the appropriate use of sleeping pills to treat insomnia.

Many people believe that sleeping pills are overused, but research has shown that this is a misconception. For example, survey data have shown that benzodiazepine hypnotics are actually used very conservatively. A recent telephone survey of individuals who took these medications revealed that the majority (74 percent) had not used them continuously for more than fourteen days at a time. *Sixty-four percent of the people surveyed took fewer than thirty doses of sleep medication per year.* And only 11 percent of the sample reported using the medication nightly for longer than twelve months.

While sleeping pills are not as overprescribed or overused as many people think, the decision to take *any* medication should be made thoughtfully because sleeping pills, like all other drugs, have both benefits and risks.

ARE SLEEPING PILLS FOR YOU?

If you have insomnia, you should keep a sleep log, establish your bed- and rise time, apply the ten tips for better sleep, and if necessary try one or more of the behavioral therapies in the preceding chapter. At the same time, you may also wish to use a sleeping pill. Sleeping pills can be used alone but will probably work best when combined with other techniques. Your chances of lasting success will be far greater if you build your sleep program step-by-step and use sleeping pills in the context of the overall program.

Talk to your doctor about sleeping pill options. You and your doctor together should make the decision for you to use a sleeping pill, whether the medication used will be a prescription or over-the-counter drug. Talking to your doctor is particularly important if you are taking any medications for another health problem or if you have any physical or mental disorder.

How do you feel about the prospect of using a sleeping pill? Many people appreciate the option of a medication to help them fall asleep faster and stay asleep longer. The knowledge that the pill will help to conquer their insomnia when it's needed is a great comfort to them. Other people dislike the idea of using any medication or artificial substance to help them sleep. The notion of putting something foreign in their bodies is unpleasant to them. Some may even feel that using medication is a sign of failure.

Whether you are comfortable, uncomfortable, or uncertain about the use of sleeping pills, there are some important factors to consider if you want to determine whether sleeping pills might help you. Answer yes or no:

1. Consider the severity of your nighttime symptoms of insomnia.
   a. Are your insomnia symptoms intolerable (i.e., do you feel you have reached the end of your rope in dealing with this problem)?
   b. Are your insomnia symptoms severe?
2. Consider the severity of your daytime symptoms of insomnia.
   a. Are you fatigued or sleepy during the day?
   b. Is your fatigue or sleepiness making it difficult for you to function in your usual activities at work or at home?
   c. Is your fatigue or sleepiness placing yourself or others in danger?

If you answered yes to any question (especially 2c), you may be a candidate for the use of a sleeping pill.

Once you have determined whether you are a candidate for medication, you need to consider the type of insomnia that you have and the features of the various drugs that are available. Many formulations exist, and not everyone can take all types. Again, I strongly advise you to discuss your decision to use any type of sleeping pill with your doctor. Be sure to share any details about your situation that will affect the type of pill you can take. For example, is there any possibility that you are pregnant? Do you consume alcohol? Are you taking any other sedating medications? Answers to questions like these will help you and your doctor make the best choices.

PEOPLE WHO SHOULD AVOID SLEEPING PILLS OR USE THEM WITH CAUTION

Group	Reasons	Comments
Children and adolescents younger than age eighteen.	Behavioral techniques often work very well.	Benzodiazepine sleeping pills are not recommended for children with insomnia.
Pregnant women and nursing mothers.	The drug may reach the developing fetus through the placenta or the nursing infant through breast milk.	Although sleeping pills are not strictly prohibited for use at this time, it is best to avoid all drugs, as testing has been minimal.
People with a history of alcohol abuse or drug abuse.	Benzodiazepines and non-benzodiazepine hypnotics pose a greater risk of dependence or addiction in this group.	Behavioral treatments and other types of sleep aids can be used without great risk of abuse. Consult your doctor.
People with sleep-related disorders including sleep apnea.	Some medications make arousal or breathing difficult and could therefore pose a danger to people with sleep apnea or sleep disorders.	Don't take sleep aids without consulting your doctor.
People who must be able to awaken quickly (e.g., firefighters, parents caring for an infant).	Some sleeping pills can cause disorientation or mental impairment if the person is awakened during the sleep period.	Be sure to tell your doctor about your situation; he or she may be able to select a suitable drug.

What Kind of Insomnia Do You Have?

The appropriateness of sleeping pills also depends on the type of insomnia you have.

The first category is *transient insomnia*, which lasts up to a few days. It's commonly a response to a short-term stress. Any of us might experience a physical or emotional stress such as the loss of a loved one or a family pet, financial difficulties, hospitalization, or arguments with a spouse. Joyous occasions can be stressful, too: the night before a trip, a wedding, or a graduation. Even changes in your sleep environment can contribute to transient insomnia: sleeping in a strange environment (e.g., a hotel room), noise, light, and uncomfortable temperature or humidity conditions. Transient insomnia can be effectively treated with a one-two punch: resolving or relieving the acute stress and using a hypnotic medication on the few nights when insomnia is present. It might seem that if insomnia is going to go away in a few days anyway, you could just wait it out. However, excessive daytime sleepiness can pose dangers to you, and you also run the risk of starting a nighttime pattern that will continue.

Recurrent transient insomnia is transient insomnia that periodically recurs. For example, a sales representative who travels out of town to her home office each month experiences insomnia on the night that she spends in her hotel room. The stress of preparing to leave home, traveling, and being at the main office, as well as the environmental stress of being in an unusual sleep environment, may all contribute to her difficulty sleeping. Each month, she endures these one or two nights of insomnia. In this case, she should be encouraged to try to deal with the stressful situation by changing her sleep habits, but hypnotic medication might be recommended for the nights that she spends away from home.

The second type, *short-term insomnia*, lasts from several days to several weeks. Again the cause is often stress, but environmental, medical, or emotional problems may also play a part. The goal of the treatment is often to resolve the underlying cause, but the addition of a hypnotic medication, especially with behavioral techniques, can help provide early relief. This strategy assumes that the person is a fairly normal or good sleeper who is experiencing a bad episode of insomnia and will return to the previous pattern of sleeping with effective short-term treatment. The medication may be taken nightly for a short time and then gradually tapered off and discontinued. The medication is given to reduce the chance the insomnia will become chronic.

The third category, *chronic insomnia*, lasts from several weeks to months or even years. While a number of factors may start it (stress, environmental factors, medical illness, psychiatric illness, alcohol or substance abuse), perpetuating factors are almost always at work, such as poor sleep habits, conditioning, or irrational beliefs about sleep. For this reason, good sleep habits and behavioral therapy are critical as a complement to medication treatment. You can use the medicine a variety of ways. Sleeping pills may be used along with the behavioral program. Some people respond well to taking medication nightly for extended periods. Others work with their doctors to establish an effective intermittent dosing schedule. For example, the person might take the sleeping pill on Friday through Sunday nights, but go without it the rest of the week. Finally, some people with chronic insomnia use medication only on nights when their symptoms are particularly bad.

Will I Get Hooked?

If you and your doctor are considering sleeping pills as part of your sleep program, you may be worrying that you will become dependent on the medication. Actually, this outcome is not likely. You and your doctor can take some easy steps to maximize the benefits and minimize any risks. If you have tended to be fearful about the use of a pill, talk to your doctor about possible risks and benefits, so you can make an informed decision.

Dependence can be physical, psychological, or both. In *physical dependence*, the drug changes your body in such a way that you crave the drug. In *psychological dependence*, you believe you need the drug, but no physical need exists. If dependence on sleeping pills does occur, it usually does so after *long-term, nightly use*.

If you are physically dependent on some types of sleeping pills, your insomnia may return when you reduce or discontinue the medication. This is known as *rebound insomnia*. If you miss a dose or stop the medication suddenly, you also may experience withdrawal symptoms including sweating, clamminess, cravings, mood changes, depression, headaches, nervousness or anxiety, convulsions, tremors, and abdominal and muscle cramps. Rebound insomnia and withdrawal symptoms are not only unpleasant but also may lead you to resume drug use. You might feel that you "can't sleep without medication" and not be inclined to discontinue the drug. If you develop this kind of psychological dependence, remember that appropriately discontinuing the medication will reduce the chance of rebound insomnia and withdrawal symptoms. To avoid such symptoms, don't stop using a drug abruptly. Instead, ask your doctor about a schedule for tapering off your dose gradually.

When some sleeping pills are taken for an extended time, they grow less effective. When *drug tolerance* develops, a dosage that helped at first no longer produces the desired results. Increasing your dose may or may not work, and it is not always wise. Tolerance to sleeping pills usually develops after a period of nightly or frequent use. The situation is less likely if you take your medication as prescribed by your doctor.

Despite all these dire warnings, while dependence is possible, it's not likely. Research has shown overwhelmingly that most people who use sleep medications don't become dependent upon them and don't become addicted for three good reasons. First, today's sleep medicines include new drugs that are safer and seem less likely to cause dependence than those of the past. Second, many people are aware of the potential for dependence and use the proper precautions. Finally, most doctors are also cautious about sleep medications and will carefully monitor your use. So if you and your doctor are discussing the possibility that a sleeping pill will help you, don't let an unfounded fear of "getting hooked" keep you from getting the relief you need.

HOW TO TAKE SLEEPING PILLS

If you have decided to use a sleeping pill, there are ways to ensure that you get the maximum benefit. To think that a medication will work no matter what you do is unrealistic. You have to set the stage for success.

- **Use behavioral methods while you are using sleeping pills.** Behavioral methods will increase the chance of a positive response and will also help resolve the underlying source of the insomnia. In a recent survey, 69 percent of sleep specialists said they believed a combination of medication and behavioral therapy was a very effective treatment for short-term insomnia, and more than 50 percent believed that this combination was the most effective treatment for chronic insomnia. Use sleeping pills in the context of a complete sleep program: maintain a regular bedtime and rise time, avoid naps, get regular exercise, create a comfortable sleep environment, follow a presleep routine, schedule worry time that is separate from your sleeping time, and so on.

- **Take your sleeping pill before bedtime.** About fifteen to thirty minutes before bedtime is best, unless your prescription states otherwise. Some of the newer medications, such as Ambien, should be taken right as you go to sleep. If you don't take your sleeping pill before bed, but realize that you're having a problem with insomnia and might need one, avoid tossing and turning for too long before taking the pill. Your insomnia can develop a froth if you allow it to stir around for too long, and it can then be more difficult for the pill to take effect. It may not work at all.

- **Ask your doctor whether you should take a pill in the middle of the night.** If you occasionally awaken during the night and can't get back to sleep, should you take a pill then? The answer depends on the time of night and the medication. Some sleep medications produce daytime sleepiness if taken too late into the night, while others don't. If you *routinely* have insomnia during the night or wake up too early (maintenance or terminal insomnia), there are medications that you can take at the beginning of the night that will help keep you asleep during the night.

- **Take your pill on an empty stomach.** That way, the medication will be absorbed more quickly and will begin to work faster. Besides food, avoid medications that slow down the stomach's action, such as antacids containing aluminum.

- **Take the prescribed dose.** Resist the impulse to be creative with your dose or schedule and take your medication as prescribed. If you reduce the dosage (e.g., by cutting the pill in half), it may not work. Taking more medication later that same night may not help and could make things worse. Give the medication a chance to work. Insomnia that has gone on for months may not be overcome in the first or second night on a sleeping pill.

- **Reduce the chance of drug interactions.** Most sleeping pills are generally safe when taken with other drugs. However, you should be cautious about taking sleeping pills when you are taking a medication that suppresses the activity of the central nervous system (such as antianxiety medication). In general, you can protect yourself against drug interactions by knowing the names, purposes, and strengths of all your medications. Read the labels and package inserts so that you understand how to take the medicine and can take the proper precautions. When you are taking a sleeping medication, talk to your doctor before taking any new medication. Keeping track of your medications is especially important if you are seeing specialists as well as a primary care provider (family physician or internist). Your primary care provider should be aware of what your oncologist, rheumatologist, urologist, gynecologist, or other specialist prescribes, but communication between busy medical offices is not always timely or smooth. Some people overcome confusion by tossing all of their medication bottles into a paper bag when they go for an office visit. Others keep a written record in a diary or on an index card that they carry in a wallet. Whatever method you choose, be aware that you play a key role in protecting yourself against drug interactions.

• **Avoid alcohol on nights that you take a sleeping pill.** Alcohol is a sedative, but it doesn't help you sleep. Not only can alcohol worsen your sleep, but it can interact with some sleeping pills in dangerous and potentially lethal ways. Also, avoid caffeine and nicotine, which are stimulants.

• **Don't use the medication excessively.** Don't use sleep medication excessively. While the risks associated with sleeping pills is minimal, it's best to follow the motto "less is more." If you need the medication nightly, and this is what was prescribed, by all means take it nightly. But if you think that you can get by with intermittent or as-needed use, talk with your doctor. The less frequently you use a sleep medication, the more likely it is to be powerful on the nights that you do take it.

SLEEP MEDICATIONS
Benzodiazepine Hypnotics

The most common prescription drugs for insomnia are benzodiazepines, which can be useful for transient, short-term, or chronic sleep

Much Better Than in the Past

Sleep-promoting substances have been used throughout history. Until this century, most were created from herbs and other natural ingredients, but the term natural *doesn't necessarily mean "harmless." Today's prescription sleep aids are a vast improvement over some of the potions used in the past.*

- *The Victorians routinely used laudanum, a tincture of opium, which is a powerful narcotic painkiller that induces a trance or sleep. Working mothers often dosed their infants so they'd sleep while the mothers were at work, with harmful and sometimes fatal results.*

- *Town chemists and traveling patent-medicine salesmen once sold tonics for the treatment of insomnia; the most abundant, and possibly the only sleep-promoting, ingredient was alcohol.*

- *During the middle and late nineteenth century, widely used treatments for insomnia included chloral hydrate ("knockout drops" or "mickeys"—what the bad guy slips into m'lady's drink in murder mysteries) and bromides (central nervous system depressants that are now out of favor because of their side effects).*

- *Barbiturates were first used at the turn of the century. Barbital and phenobarbital were used widely for many years, but the potential for addiction and fatal overdose led to their decline.*

- *Other drugs freely prescribed in the fifties and sixties (Placidyl, Quaaludes, and others) carry many of the same risks as barbiturates and are now almost never prescribed for insomnia.*

problems. They have relatively low rates of adverse effects, don't interact with many other commonly used drugs, and are generally safe if an accidental overdose occurs. The effectiveness of benzodiazepine hypnotics has been documented by hundreds of clinical tests. These medicines result in a significant decrease in time to sleep onset and an increase in sleep efficiency, and their users report that sleep quality is good. They do reduce delta (deep) stages of sleep.

No evidence shows that any one benzodiazepine hypnotic is better than any other, but differences exist among the drugs. Some may induce sleep more rapidly than others when taken in a single dose, some may work best when taken over a few consecutive days, and some have fewer side effects.

Some benzodiazepine drugs act over many hours, which can lead to drowsiness the next day. If you suffer only from sleep-onset insomnia, a benzodiazepine that enters the bloodstream rapidly and remains only a short time would be a good choice. Since the drug will be distributed, metabolized, and eliminated over a short time, it shouldn't alter your sleep when you don't need it. On the other hand, if you suffer from sleep maintenance or terminal insomnia, you may need a drug that remains in the body for an intermediate or long time. In this case, you will have an adequate amount of the drug in your body over a sufficient period of time to help you stay asleep through the sleep period. When you and your doctor are choosing a benzodiazepine drug for you, consider whether it is a "short acting" or "long acting" medication.

✳☾✳☾✳☾✳☾✳☾✳☾✳☾✳

Duration of Benzodiazepines

Generic Name	Trade Name	Speed of Onset	Usual Duration of Action
Alprazolam	Xanax	Moderate	Intermediate
Diazepam	Valium	Rapid	Long
Estazolam	Prosom	Moderate	Intermediate
Flurazepam	Dalmane	Rapid	Long
Lorazepam	Ativan	Moderate	Intermediate
Quazepam	Doral	Rapid	Intermediate
Temazepam	Restoril	Slow	Intermediate
Traizolam	Halcion	Moderate	Short

Long-term use of benzodiazepine drugs may cause physical and psychological dependence. Your health care provider can markedly reduce any likelihood that you will experience these problems by carefully managing your use of sleeping pills; however, you must do your part by remaining aware of the potential risk, using the medication only as prescribed, and promptly reporting any difficulties. Abruptly stopping a benzodiazepine hypnotic, particularly the short-acting agents, can cause withdrawal symptoms including a general feeling of malaise, mild mood disturbance, anxiety or apprehension, irritability, dizziness, and decreased appetite. It can also cause rebound insomnia and make you feel jittery, wide awake, and unable to sleep. Rebound insomnia can be more severe than your insomnia used to be. To prevent such withdrawal symptoms, you have to taper off your use gradually.

Zolpidem (Ambien)

Released just a few years ago, zolpidem, sold under the trade name Ambien, is now widely prescribed for insomnia and has even been approved for use on the space shuttle. Zolpidem is an imidazopyridine, which is different from conventional benzodiazepine hypnotics. Unlike benzodiazepines, it does not seem to reduce delta sleep, so sleep architecture remains closer to normal. Zolpidem reduces time to sleep onset, makes it easier to fall asleep, increases total sleep time, and decreases the number of awakenings during the sleep period. It appears effective in transient, short-term, and chronic insomnia. Although the drug is cleared from the bloodstream rather quickly, it has helped people who have trouble staying asleep, too.

In one 1994 study, Drs. Martin Scharf, Thomas Roth, Gerald Vogel, and James Walsh found that Ambien was effective for longer than four weeks of nightly administration. Another study found continued effectiveness for several months.

Zolpidem also has potential advantages over benzodiazepines:
- The risks of tolerance, dependence, and withdrawal symptoms seem to be less.
- Sleep laboratory tests have shown that discontinuation after several consecutive nights of use does not result in rebound insomnia.
- It is usually not associated with next-day sedation, memory impairment, or slips and falls in the elderly.

• Unlike benzodiazepines, zolpidem does not depress respiration, offering a potential advantage for people with breathing disorders.

Side effects, which are rare, can include drowsiness, dizziness, and diarrhea. Older people are a bit more likely to experience a side effect, particularly a headache or drowsiness. Zolpidem should be avoided if you are pregnant or nursing.

If you are using a benzodiazepine hypnotic but want to try zolpidem, you must consult with your doctor to develop a plan for tapering off and discontinuing the benzodiazepine hypnotic.

Another non-benzodiazepine hypnotic is now in the trial stage. Whereas it has not yet been approved in the United States, it shows great promise. It affects the brain similarly to Zolpidem, has less risk of tolerance and dependence than with benzodiazepine drugs, and has very few next-day effects.

Sedating Antidepressants

Although a benzodiazepine or non-benzodiazepine hypnotic medication is the treatment of choice, a secondary option is a sedating antidepressant. If your physician recommends an antidepressant as a sleep aid, it's not necessarily because he or she suspects you of being depressed. While antidepressants are primarily used to improve mood in people with depression, a side effect is sedation. Clinical experience suggests that, taken before bed, they can promote sleep onset and maintain sleep, though there is little scientific data to prove their general effectiveness in treating insomnia. The most sedating antidepressants are amitriptyline (Elavil), clomipramine (Anafranil), doxepin (Adapin, Sinequan), and trazodone (Desyrel).

A sedating antidepressant may be the drug of choice if the person has experienced side effects, tolerance, or dependence with benzodiazepine hypnotics; has both insomnia and depression; has a history of alcohol or drug problems; or has health problems that preclude the use of a benzodiazepine.

There is no risk of dependence with an antidepressant. However, the medication may become ineffective after only a few days or weeks. Potential side effects include blurred vision, low blood pressure, rapid heart beat, irregular heart beat, dry mouth, constipation, urinary retention, and impairments in sexual functioning. If your

✳ ☾ ✳ ☾ ✳ ☾ ✳ ☾ ✳ ☾ ✳ ☾ ✳ ☾ ✳

Sedating and Alerting Antidepressants

Some antidepressant medications are sedating, and others are stimulating. The "alerting" medications not only fail to help resolve insomnia but also may be the underlying cause if taken for another health problem.

SEDATING

amitriptyline (Elavil)
clomipramine (Anafranil)
doxepin (Adapin, Sinequan)
trazodone (Desyrel)

ALERTING

bupropion (Wellbutrin)
fluoxetine (Prozac)
isocarboxazid (Marplan)
phenelzine (Nardil)
tranylcypromine (Parnate)
venlafaxine (Effexor)

doctor prescribes a sedating antidepressant and it fails to work, stops working, or produces unwanted side effects, don't hesitate to call your doctor.

Antihistamines

Sometimes used as sleep aids are antihistimines. Besides helping with allergies, these drugs also have a sedating effect, which has led to their occasional use as sleep aids.

The most sedating antihistamines are chlorpheniramine (Chlor-Trimeton), diphenhydramine (Benadryl), hydroxazine (Atarax), and promethazine (Phenergan). Such antihistamines are believed to decrease time to sleep onset and decrease REM sleep time in healthy people. Some antihistamines require a prescription, but low doses of Benadryl and Chlor-Trimeton are available without one.

Only a few studies of the use of sedating antihistamines in the treatment of insomnia have been conducted. In one study, Drs. Kudo and Kurihara in Tokyo, Japan, found a good response among psychiatric patients with insomnia who were given the antihistamine diphenhydramine (Benadryl) in doses of 12.5 to 50 mg. More than 60 percent of the people in this study reported at least slight improvement after treatment for two weeks. But not all studies show positive results with antihistamines.

There are some caveats regarding the use of antihistamines in the treatment of insomnia. First, some antihistamines are not sedative at all. These are the "second generation" antihistamine medications such as terfenadine (Seldane), loratadine (Claritin), and astemizole (Hisminal). Second, many sleep specialists don't recommend sedating antihistamines because laboratory evidence of their effectiveness in insomnia is so sparse. The sedation experienced with some antihistamines may not be sufficient to reduce time to sleep onset in insomnia, and it's not clear if the sedation is sufficient to sustain sleep. Even if an antihistamine is helpful initially, it may lose its effectiveness in a matter of days.

Antihistamines can also be associated with significant side effects, most commonly dizziness, disturbed coordination; gastric distress; thickening of bronchial secretions; and dryness of the mouth, nose, and throat. A number of other, less common side effects are also possible. Sedation may carry over to the next day and impair performance. These side effects are more significant than those of the traditional benzodiazepine and non-benzodiazepine hypnotics.

Nonprescription Sleep Aids

Many nonprescription medications are marketed as sleep aids. About 40 percent of people with insomnia have tried one. Compoz, Nytol, and Sominex contain diphenhydramine, and Unisom contains doxylamine. Both diphenhydramine and doxylamine are sedating antihistamines, so they may or may not be effective for you. More than half the people who use these products have a residual hangover effect the next day. You may have already tried an over-the-counter medicine and had a good response with no significant adverse reaction. If you failed to get relief, however, you have lots of company.

Dr. Wallace Mendelson of the University of Chicago Sleep Laboratory recently reported on a long-term, follow-up study of people with insomnia. He found that while rates of over-the-counter sleeping pill use go up over time, there is a low rate of satisfaction with them.

Over-the-counter drugs are most effective for occasional sleep problems, rather than long-term insomnia.

We tend to think of over-the-counter products as without complications—if they weren't, why would they be available without a prescription? But over-the-counter sleep aids containing antihistamines may cause a variety of side effects, including dry mouth and constipation. You may have fewer adverse reactions from some prescription hypnotic medication than from over-the-counter preparations.

Also usually contained in some over-the-counter sleep aids is scopolamine, which reduces the activity of the central nervous system. In low doses, scopolamine is known to produce drowsiness, fatigue, and amnesia, and it's also known to reduce REM sleep. Among its adverse effects can be dry mouth, blurred vision, urinary retention, and constipation.

In the past few years, manufacturers of over-the-counter pain medications have become aware that nighttime pain can be a source of disturbed sleep. These manufacturers have combined pain relievers with mild sleep aids. Among these medications are Unisom with Pain Relief, Tylenol PM, and Excedrin PM, all of which contain some combination of the antihistamine diphenhydramine and acetaminophen. These pain and sleep aids have not been extensively studied, but may be quite helpful to people who suffer from a combination of nighttime discomfort and insomnia.

"NATURAL" SLEEP AIDS

"Natural" sleep aids are herbs, hormones, or other substances found naturally in plants or foods. Most are not proven effective, and some are potentially dangerous. Unlike prescription or nonprescription medication, they have not been through the FDA testing and approving procedure. Lack of standards or quality control can lead to problems. In this case, "natural" doesn't necessarily mean "pure" or "harmless."

Tryptophan

Trypotophan is an amino acid that is found naturally in many foods, including meat, milk, fish, poultry, cheese, eggs, and some vegetables. It's one of the substances that our bodies use to make protein, and it's a natural precursor to the neurotransmitter serotonin, which is involved in the production of sleep. Some time ago, researchers learned that by increasing levels of tryptophan, you can increase levels of serotonin in the brain, and this effect promotes sleep in both animals and humans. These findings led to interest in the use of tryptophan as a treatment for insomnia.

Since tryptophan is a natural substance and not a drug, it was quickly and widely promoted by health food stores as a "natural sleep aid," available in capsule or tablet form. People using tryptophan for sleep would take their pills before going to bed, much like they would use a sleeping pill. It was used this way without problem for many years. Suddenly, in the late 1980s, clinicians began seeing a group of serious symptoms in some patients: muscle pain, fatigue, weakness, skin rash, pulmonary infiltrates, and cardiac arrhythmias. The symptoms were identified as eosinophilia-myalgia syndrome, a disorder in which too many eosinophiles (white blood cells) develop. The common denominator among the people with this syndrome was that they used tryptophan. Investigations by the U.S. government revealed that a contaminant in the pills, resulting from the manufacturing process, was responsible for the problem. Since then, tryptophan sales have been banned in the United States.

Melatonin

Melatonin is all the rage. Its supporters have promoted it for just about everything that could possibly ail the human body or mind, including insomnia. Many claims for melatonin are highly questionable, including anticancer properties and extending the lifespan. Let's look at the facts.

Melatonin is a hormone that is naturally secreted by the pineal gland at night. In healthy individuals, melatonin levels are lowest during the day, increase in the evening hours just prior to sleep onset, and peak shortly after sleep onset. The hormone is thought to play an important role in organizing daily circadian rhythms. It seems to provide a biologic signal to begin nighttime behavior.

The association between melatonin and nighttime sleep has led several investigators to study the use of a melatonin supplement as a sleep aid. Studies have suggested that small amounts (0.3 mg) of melatonin may help some people fall asleep faster. Some studies have in fact found that melatonin supplements may help people adapt to jet lag and nightshift work. There is also some evidence that melatonin may be helpful in treating sleep/wake schedule disorders, such as delayed sleep phase syndrome (see chapter 8). However, despite the media's enthusiasm and the high rates of sales of melatonin supplements (now rivaling sales of vitamin C), *there is little evidence that supplementary melatonin is generally effective as a treatment for insomnia.* In fact, in some studies, participants reported that they didn't feel a bit sleepier after taking a melatonin supplement. Clearly, more research is needed before we can determine the usefulness of melatonin for anything, including insomnia.

One interesting study of melatonin was reported recently by researchers in Israel. They investigated melatonin supplements in the elderly. There have been reports that melatonin levels decline with aging and that impaired melatonin secretion is associated with disturbed sleep in the elderly. The researchers thought that "replacing" melatonin might promote better sleep. The study found that melatonin administration did shorten the time to sleep onset and increase sleep time. Also, sleep quality deteriorated following discontinuation of the melatonin. However, this study involved only a small number of people and requires further follow-up.

Many people with insomnia have tried larger amounts of melatonin (2 to 5 mg) before bedtime as a sleep aid. I do not recommend this regime. Because melatonin is a dietary supplement, not an approved medication, it has not been exposed to the rigorous product testing for effectiveness and safety that is required for prescription medication. Lack of testing exposes you to dangers like these:

- The quality of melatonin contained in the pills varies, depending on the skill, budget, and conscience of the manufacturer.
- The quantity of melatonin pills also varies. There may be dis-

crepancies between the amount stated on the label and the amount in the pill.

- A recent report showed that chemical analyses of four of six melatonin products from health food stores contained impurities that could not be characterized, which is precisely the type of problem that caused so much suffering among users of tryptophan.
- Studies have not established the proper dosage of melatonin.

Here are some more reasons to be cautious:

- Melatonin can be associated with side effects, including headache, nausea, and a fuzzy or giddy feeling.
- Melatonin constricts the coronary arteries. Its effects on people with coronary artery disease are unclear.
- People with high blood pressure have higher numbers of melatonin receptors in their cerebral arteries. We don't know what this means, but precaution is certainly warranted.
- Perhaps most important, melatonin is a hormone, not a vitamin. Hormones play complex and powerful roles, many of which are not yet fully understood. We pause and think before taking birth control pills, estrogen, or androgens. Why rush to take melatonin?

If you still think you'd like to try melatonin, or you have questions about this substance, ask your health care provider.

Herbal Remedies

Herbal remedies for insomnia have been used for centuries as nature's own cure. Chamomile is usually consumed as a tea, drunk warm shortly before bedtime. Similarly, valerian root is usually steeped into warm water to make tea but can also be dropped into water or can even be purchased in pill form. While many people swear by these substances, we have little scientific evidence that they work. Perhaps the virtue of taking a few minutes to relax and enjoy a warm beverage before bedtime is the most effective component of herbal remedies. However, if these remedies work for you, by all means, take advantage of them. There are no good reasons not to try herbal remedies, but don't be surprised if they are not effective for you.

Herbal remedies are not limited to teas. One method that has actually been studied is the use of herbs, such as lavender, to create a soothing aroma. The results suggest that aroma therapy may actually help promote rest and sleep. Another, thoroughly pleasant possibility is to have a partner smooth on oils extracted from plants and give you a wonderfully soothing massage.

✳ 8 ✳

When Your Sleep Rhythms Are Disrupted

Each of us has an internal, biological clock, called a circadian rhythm, that makes us feel sleepy at regular times each day, and stop sleeping at regular times, too. Your circadian rhythm helps you sleep regularly and sufficiently. As we discussed in chapter 4, the circadian rhythm takes its cues from the environment, particularly light, but is powerful enough to influence sleep timing even when external time cues are missing. It even prevails when sleep is disturbed by medical, psychiatric, or certain sleep disorders.

However, a person's circadian rhythm can be disrupted, which in turn disrupts patterns of sleepiness and awakening. When this happens, the timing of sleepiness is no longer in sync with the times you want to sleep.

Circadian rhythm problems can have external causes, most commonly shift work and high-speed air travel across time zones. They can also be caused by sleep disorders that cause sleep to occur earlier than you'd like (*phase advanced*), later (*phase delayed*), irregularly, or at intervals other than twenty-four hours. Disrupted circadian rhythms can cause significant symptoms, including psychological problems, and can impair mental, social, or occupational functioning. For example, someone with a phase delay is likely to have difficulty getting up for work in the morning, and when awakened, may be mentally sluggish early in the day.

In this chapter, you will learn ways to cope with circadian rhythm sleep disorders, whether they have been caused by your night shifts at work or by a slip in your body's internal watch.

SHIFT WORK

Shift work is scheduled outside regular daytime work hours (nine to five). It includes evening and night work, rotating shifts, split shifts, and extended hours. The most common kind of shift work is a regular schedule of *evening* or *night work*, such as 3:00 P.M. to 11:00 P.M. or 11:00 P.M. to 7:00 A.M., five days a week with a two-day interruption. *Rotating shifts* change periodically; for example, an employee may work days for several weeks, then evenings for several weeks, then nights, and then rotate back to days. *Split-shift* workers do all or part of one shift, take a planned break, and then work all or part of the next shift. *Extended-hours* employees work longer than a usual work day, sometimes more than twelve hours a day.

Shift work is far more prevalent than most people realize. It's quite common in transportation industries (air, rail, shipping, trucking), medicine, law enforcement, fire protection, the postal service, the military, manufacturing, entertainment, finance, and hotel and restaurant management. Even your local bakery employs shift workers to bake through the night so the breads and pastries are fresh the next morning. Special circumstances, such as a storm that brings power lines down, may suddenly turn workers used to a daytime schedule into shift workers or extended-shift workers.

In fact, about one in six people in the American workforce is involved in some form of shift work. About 16 percent of full-time employees regularly do shift work (18 percent of the men and 13 percent of the women). At least one spouse does shift work in one-quarter of dual-earner families with children. Of these enormous numbers of people, only one-quarter *choose* shift work. Three-quarters accept these schedules because they are a job requirement. Instinctively, people avoid shift work because they recognize the stress of being out of sync with their biological rhythm and with the schedule followed by most of society.

Shift work can disrupt sleep and lead to sleep deprivation, fatigue, and sleepiness. In turn, sleep deprivation often makes it harder for workers to cope with other stresses caused by shift work, for example, the strain on a marriage when a husband and wife work different hours.

Shift-work schedules sometimes demand that a person remain awake, alert, and functioning at a time that is normally reserved for rest or sleep. Consequently, sleep must take place during hours that are usually reserved for other activities, which causes problems because the worker's internal circadian rhythm and the demands of the external world clash. The worker experiences fatigue and sleepiness during waking hours and difficulty sleeping during the hours reserved for sleep. Soon the worker may experience feelings of general sleep deprivation; physical complaints (most commonly digestive problems); and reduced attention, memory, and concentration.

Some people can adjust to a shift work schedule without too much difficulty, but others find it intolerable. If you simply can't adjust to shift work, you're better off seeking employment that does not require work outside of normal hours. If you choose to be involved in shift work, or your career offers no options, here are some ways you can cope.

Coping with Evening and Night Shifts

At first, just about everyone has some difficulty adjusting to evening or night shifts. Here are ways to smooth your transition and realign your circadian rhythm with your work-imposed sleep schedule.

- Make every effort to maintain a regular sleep schedule with a set bedtime and rise time and sufficient time for sleep. For example, if you work the evening shift and return home just after midnight and you need eight hours of sleep, you could set your regular bedtime at two A.M. and your regular rise time at ten A.M.
- Keep your bedtime and rise time relatively constant, even on weekends.
- If you must shorten your sleep period, use a "preventive" nap before going in for your work shift.
- Be strict about reserving your sleep period just for sleep.
- Turn down the ringer on your phone at bedtime. Train your

friends and relatives to call at appropriate hours by not answering the phone just before or during your sleep time. Let an answering machine or voice mail pick up your calls.

- Adjust your patterns of socialization, household chores and errands, meal times, phone calls, and so on to be consistent with your work and sleep schedule. Avoid eating a heavy breakfast just before going to bed and don't interrupt your daytime sleep period for lunch.
- While caffeine can help you sustain alertness during an evening or night shift, avoid it in the hours just before bed.

If you work a night shift, the problems experienced by William may well seem familiar. When he came to the sleep center, William had been working nights at a plastics manufacturing plant for four months. His shift was eleven P.M. to seven A.M. beginning Sunday night and ending Friday morning. Over the prior months, when he returned home about 7:30, he helped the children get ready for schoool, then he enjoyed a cup of coffee and quick breakfast with his wife before she left for her job. Once alone, William felt a bit "wired" and would take some time to relax or even to run errands. He went to bed around ten A.M. and slept through until about five P.M., getting up just before his wife returned home from work. William's sleep was occasionally interrupted by noise, light, or the commotion created by the children after they returned home from school. He spent his evenings with his family before leaving for work about 10:30.

William found the schedule tolerable during the work week, but the weekends were increasingly difficult. After getting off of work on Friday morning, he often felt full of energy. He had trouble sleeping, and in fact tried to stay awake in the hope that he would be able to fall asleep at the same time as his wife and children on Friday night, and then be with them during the day on Saturday and Sunday. However, William found it very difficult to sleep on Friday and Saturday nights and felt worn out on Saturdays and Sundays. As the weeks passed, William started to sleep poorly all the time and was always suffering from fatigue. He came to the Sleep Disorders Institute for evaluation and treatment.

I believed the root of his problem was his irregular sleep schedule, with daytime sleep during the week and nighttime sleep on the weekends. Also, William was using coffee at inappropriate times, either to help him stay awake or because of old habits (e.g., coffee in the morning with his wife). I recommended that William adopt a regular schedule of daytime sleep in order to accommodate his work schedule. He began going to bed at ten A.M. and rising at five P.M. *every day.* He no longer drank coffee before bedtime. After only a few weeks of his regular schedule, William found that he was sleeping better, feeling more refreshed upon awakening, and not suffering from sleepiness when he was awake. Because his mood was better, he was even enjoying time with his family more. After everything got back on track, William found that he could modify his sleep schedule slightly on occasion by going to bed a little bit later or rising a little bit later, and using a brief nap prior to going into work to help him feel good throughout his nighttime shift. It took some time for William to accommodate to his new schedule, but he says he feels better and is much happier with his new lifestyle.

Coping with Rotating Shifts

Rotating shifts are just plain brutal. Unfortunately, some jobs require them. This type of schedule is harder to cope with than a regular evening or night schedule because your internal circadian rhythm has to shift along with your changing work schedule. If you work rotating shifts, follow all of the same strategies as the evening or night worker and add these few strategies.

- Adjusting to rotating shifts is easier when they move clockwise, that is from days to evenings to nights. If you can, avoid rotating shifts that move counterclockwise (nights to evenings to days) or that change erratically.
- Longer periods between schedule changes make adapting easier. Try to remain on one shift for more than one week before moving to the next shift.
- Minimize stress during the days just after a rotation by avoiding situations that are physically or emotionally draining for you.

Coping with Split Shifts or Extended Hours

In split shifts and extended hours, you may be occasionally or regularly asked to work long days. Not surprisingly, as the work day lengthens, fatigue increases and productivity declines. If you're faced with this situation, these strategies may help.

- Follow the rules for evening and night shift workers, maintaining a regular sleep schedule and allowing yourself adequate time to sleep.
- If your work schedule threatens to reduce the amount of time that you can make available for sleep, consider shifting your sleep schedule. For example, if extended hours make you go to bed later than you would otherwise, plan to get up later each day.
- If your work schedule has reduced the amount of sleep you've had, try "power napping." During those long work days, take a fifteen- to thirty-minute break and nap. Power napping is especially practical for split-shift workers who have breaks built into their schedules.

JET LAG

People who travel at high speed across multiple time zones often experience jet lag, which sleep specialists call time-zone change syndrome. Upon reaching the destination, the traveler has trouble sleeping at the times appropriate in the new place, has poor or disrupted sleep, and is fatigued or sleepy when awake. Jet lag makes people irritable, alters mood, and makes it difficult to concentrate and focus on mental tasks. Many people have digestive problems like stomach cramps or discomfort, gas, constipation, and diarrhea. Jet lag is the result of the clash between the individual's internal circadian rhythm of sleep and wakefulness and the external time cues in the new time zone. It can be exacerbated by having to eat food that you wouldn't normally eat, in strange places, at times that are off your regular schedule, and in the company of people you may not even know. Consider that disrupting your circadian rhythm affects not only when you want to sleep and awaken but also the biological rhythms linked to that cycle, including body temperature and hormone secretion.

Most people find jet lag a minor inconvenience that passes in a few days. Others have severe symptoms, especially sleepiness or fatigue, that can last for more than a week. The prevalence of jet lag is not known, although most air travelers have at least some familiarity with it. It seems that the older you get, the more likely you are to get it.

If you travel west, your internal circadian rhythm is *phase advanced* relative to local time. Your internal rhythm favors sleep onset and rise times that are *earlier than normal* in the destination time zone. An eastward flight causes a *phase-delayed* shift, with sleep and rise times that are *later than normal* for the destination time. It's easier for the body to advance the sleep pattern than to delay it, so westward travel is easier than eastward travel. The severity of the symptoms also depends, of course, on how many time zones you cross.

Let's say that you are a New Yorker who usually goes to bed at eleven P.M. and rises at seven A.M. eastern standard time (EST). If you fly to Los Angeles, you will cross three time zones and "lose" three hours. You'll be ready for sleep at eight P.M. Pacific standard time (PST), just about the time your client's cocktails are being served. At four A.M. PST, you'll probably wake up. You are phase advanced. A few days later, just about the time your body readjusts, it will be time to fly eastward, and your circadian rhythm will become phase delayed relative to local time. After recrossing three time zones and "gaining" three hours, you'll be ready to sleep at two A.M. and to get up at ten A.M. EST. Sleep onset insomnia and excessive morning or daytime sleepiness will probably plague you for two or three days. (By the way, a disturbing trend in business is to schedule meetings at distant sites to run into or through weekends, taking advantage of lower hotel and airline rates. The employees have less chance to recover from jet lag before returning to the office. Companies that don't allow employees time to recuperate end up with staff members who are too tired to do anything productive and who may actually be counterproductive if they snap at customers and make mistakes.)

In addition to crossing time zones, other aspects of travel can also cause sleep loss and sleepiness. Some people become anxious before a trip and develop insomnia before even starting out. Upon arrival, westward travelers may have evening obligations that interfere with their desire to retire early, and eastward travelers may have morning obligations that prevent sleeping late into the morning. Being short on sleep can make the symptoms of jet lag worse.

People who travel frequently across time zones may experience chronic sleep disturbances. For example, air crews on long commercial flights often divide their sleep into two periods. During a layover, crew members often experience daytime sleepiness and have poor sleep.

Aircraft passengers who do not remain in the destination time zone long enough to retrain their circadian rhythms, may experience similar problems.

Studies using EEGs have shown that, following travel across multiple time zones, sleep is fragmented and a greater percentage of light Stage 1 sleep occurs. Following flight, the duration and timing of sleep is irregular. Interestingly, though jet lag is usually thought to have its greatest effect immediately after arrival in the new time zone, the EEGs showed that subsequent nights may be disturbed even if no significant effects are seen the first night.

Aircraft-cabin conditions, not jet lag, are responsible for such post-flight symptoms as dry itching eyes, irritated nasal passages, muscle cramps, headaches, nausea, abdominal distention, swelling, and dizziness. You can reduce these problems by drinking lots of nonalcoholic, noncaffeinated beverages during the flight and by moving around periodically. Drinking alcohol immediately before, during, or after a flight may contribute to the malaise of jet lag, so when the drink cart reaches your seat, have some fruit juice or other nonalcoholic beverage. Don't use alcohol as a sedative to induce sleep during or after a flight.

Minimizing Jet Lag

Normally, the body can adjust to a new time zone within several days. It can adjust to about one and a half hours of change per day following westward flights and one hour per day following eastward flights. So after a flight from New York to Los Angeles, you'll likely readjust within two days, but you'll need three days to recuperate from the return trip.

It's remarkable that the body can normally adjust so easily to a time change. It takes its cues from sunlight, your new sleeping schedule, and other habits like mealtimes.

One way to speed your adjustment is to expose yourself to bright sunlight at certain times of the day. If you have traveled west, take a walk in the sun in the afternoon. If you traveled east, get sunshine in the early morning. This routine will help reset your circadian rhythm.

By the way, if you're going to be in a new place for only one or two days, a reasonable strategy is to just stay on your usual schedule.

Researchers are currently studying whether sleeping pills might help treat jet lag by helping the traveler fall asleep on the new schedule. However, there are no definitive answers yet, so it's best to consult with your doctor or a sleep specialist if you're considering making sleeping pills part of your solution.

Researchers—and frequent air travelers—have developed several ways to ward off the symptoms of jet lag:

- A few days before your trip, begin going to bed and getting up at or near the appropriate times for your destination time zone. Before a westbound trip, go to bed later and get up later. Before an eastbound trip, go to bed earlier and get up earlier.
- In the days prior to departure, start timing your daily routines to the new time zone. You can alter your meal times and periods of activity and rest.
- Pack items from home that might help you to sleep, such as your favorite pillow. If you usually use a white noise machine, take it along. Ear plugs and eye shades may also be helpful.
- Avoid alcohol or caffeinated beverages prior to and during travel. But do drink lots of water or fruit juice to prevent dehydration while traveling.
- To make it easier to adjust your bedtime, schedule your flight so you arrive in the afternoon or early evening and then stay awake until your desired bedtime in the new time zone. Or choose a directional strategy. When traveling west, pick a flight that arrives shortly before your bedtime. Avoid sleeping on the flight and then go to bed as soon as you arrive. When traveling east, choose a flight that arrives near your rise time. Try to sleep on the plane, start your day once you've reached your destination, and then go to bed that night at the desired bedtime.
- Avoid heavy meals during flight or just before bedtime.
- Pack a travel survival kit that includes items like chewing gum, hand and face cream, wet towelettes, nasal moisturizer spray, slippers, neck pillow, a good book, or snacks—anything that might make your trip more comfortable.
- Once you've arrived at your destination, avoid exercise just before bedtime.
- Make certain that your temporary sleep environment is conducive to sleep. The bed should be comfortable, and the room should be

quiet. The temperature and humidity of the room should also be to your liking. If anything is amiss, don't hesitate to ask for a room change.

SLEEP-PHASE DISORDERS

Do you know someone who is very definitely a "morning person"? Or very definitely a "night person" who doesn't seem to come alive until the wee hours? More than likely, this behavior is just a personal preference, but it can be a sign of a sleep-phase disorder in which the internal circadian rhythm is no longer aligned with the external environment. Unlike shift work or jet lag, this sleep problem is caused by an internal disruption of the timing mechanism within the body.

Delayed Sleep Phase Syndrome

The characteristics of delayed sleep phase syndrome are

- Sleep onset and wake times that are consistently and stubbornly later than desired.
- Sleep begins at nearly the same time each day.
- Little or no difficulty staying asleep once sleep has begun.
- The person finds it extremely difficult to wake up at the desired time in the morning.
- The person has a severe or absolute inability to move sleep to earlier hours by enforcing conventional sleep and wake times.

Though delayed sleep phase syndrome is rare, it accounts for 39 percent of all diagnoses of circadian rhythm sleep disorders. It frequently begins in childhood and may be most common in adolescents; among twelve to nineteen year olds, more than 7 percent report symptoms of this problem.

People with delayed sleep phase syndrome are typically night people who feel best and are in peak form during the late evening and night hours. However, they often complain that they can't fall asleep before two A.M. Sometimes sleep is so delayed that it comes just before it's time to get up. EEGs have shown that once the person is asleep, sleep is not interrupted. The person usually awakens spontaneously in the late morning or in the afternoon. Attempts to awaken

the person earlier with an alarm clock or other means can be successful but often fail. Consequently, individuals often adapt by finding
employment or changing their schedules so they can be absent during the morning hours. People have adapted successfully in a variety
of home, academic, and work situations. However, when such accom-
modations can't be made, sustaining employment or personal relationships can be difficult.

People with delayed sleep phase syndrome are often sleepy during
the morning hours because their circadian rhythms want them to keep
on sleeping. Also, because they have gone to bed late, they simply
will not get enough hours of sleep if they have to rise earlier than
they want to. Repeated nights of insufficient sleep can markedly increase sleepiness throughout the day. People who force themselves
to rise in order to meet social or occupational obligations often suffer from sleepiness, fatigue, impaired memory and concentration, and
diminished productivity, especially in the hours just after awakening.
Many people seek professional help when they are having severe
problems functioning during the day or when they are in danger of
losing their jobs.

Delayed sleep phase syndrome is not the same thing as insomnia.
Unlike people with insomnia, people with delayed sleep phase syndrome often get normal amounts of sleep and sleep continuously and
undisturbed. They simply have a chronic and stable pattern of sleep
delay. Conventional treatments for insomnia, including sedative-
hypnotic medication, will not help. Sleep logs are important tools to
distinguish delayed sleep phase syndrome from insomnia.

Delayed sleep phase syndrome is also not the same thing as choosing to remain awake late into the night to work or play. People with
this syndrome don't have a choice. They can't get to sleep earlier, no
matter what they do. Nevertheless, some people do report that their
difficulties began after a period in which they stayed awake late at
night. University students who fall into a pattern of late night television viewing and studying, delayed bedtime and rise time, and afternoon or evening classes can experience serious difficulty when daytime
job opportunities arise or when new class schedules require morning
attendance. Shift work and seasonal changes in the light exposure can
also contribute to the development of this syndrome.

Some people with delayed sleep phase syndrome also have depression. It's not clear whether delayed sleep phase syndrome gives rise to depression or the other way around.

Tragically, delayed sleep phase syndrome is often not recognized, and others unfairly view the person as lazy, unmotivated, or mentally ill. In reality, it is a problem not of character or emotional health, but of an organ within the brain's hypothalamus, the suprachismatic nucleus. This organ, only the size of a pin, plays a key role in maintaining circadian rhythms. Research is continuing into the causes of this disorder.

Advanced Sleep Phase Syndrome

People with advanced sleep phase syndrome are morning people. Their sleep period occurs earlier than desired or acceptable. The syndrome is characterized by a stubborn, chronic inability to delay the onset of evening sleep or extend sleep later into the morning hours by enforcing conventional bedtimes and rise times.

People with this syndrome typically retire before nine P.M. and awaken between three o'clock and five A.M. They usually have difficulty functioning in the evening. If unable to retire at the usual bedtime, they may fall asleep despite their best efforts, especially in quiet, sedentary situations. They may adapt by avoiding social or other activities in the evening. Although advanced sleep phase syndrome appears to be rare, it may escape the professional attention it needs because the necessary adaptations are socially acceptable and the functional impairments associated with this disorder are not as public as in delayed sleep phase syndrome.

The sleeper awakens early, feeling fully alert, and is unable to return to sleep even when conditions favor continued sleep. Some people find early morning awakenings are frustrating and feel that they are out of step with the rest of the world. Others fill the early morning hours with productive activity. They may consider their ability to rise early to be an asset. They can be the first to arrive at work in the morning or can accomplish many tasks before others start their day.

A person who wakes up early may believe he or she has terminal insomnia. Unlike the person with insomnia, however, a person with advanced sleep phase syndrome does not have trouble staying asleep. Also, when the bedtime is delayed, early morning awakenings persist, which shows that the problem is one of timing rather than the ability to sustain sleep. However, early morning awakenings are a well-known sign of depression, so you may need the assistance of a sleep expert or your health care professional to determine the source of your problem.

Older people often have a sleep pattern of retiring and awakening earlier than younger or middle-aged adults. People who rise at four in the morning and fall asleep in the evening by 8:30 can have trouble scheduling social and family activities and can feel out of sync with the rest of society. Behavioral treatments such as going to bed later and the use of afternoon exposure to bright light can help treat phase-advanced sleep.

Sleep Rhythm Other Than Twenty-Four Hours

In a very few people, the circadian rhythm is twenty-five hours or longer. In such individuals, sleep onset and rise times are progressively delayed each day so that the sleep period is continuously moving forward. The delay of the sleep period is usually about two hours or less per day, although longer delays have been reported. The sleep period travels in and out of phase with the desired or socially acceptable hours for sleep, so that periodically—and temporarily—it's normal. Of course, this cycling can't go on for long without causing serious problems, especially difficulty sleeping at night and difficulty staying alert during the day.

Individuals with non-twenty-four-hour sleep-wake syndrome have great difficulty responding to the conventional time cues that normally shape the circadian rhythm of sleep and wakefulness. They may attempt to enforce wakefulness during the day with loud or multiple alarm clocks, caffeinated beverages, or other stimulant substances. They may attempt to induce sleep at desired times by using over-the-counter or prescription drugs, especially hypnotics, but medications cannot change the circadian rhythm. Instead of resolving the problem, these strategies, and the poor sleep habits that inevitably evolve, make the condition chronic. Some people are so frustrated by this problem, and so debilitated by sleepiness, that they give up on ever being able to synchronize their sleep to conventional hours.

Though this syndrome is rare in general, it occurs more frequently among blind persons. Three-quarters of blind people say their sleep is disturbed. A non-twenty-four-hour circadian rhythm can be the problem, as studies have shown that blind people's circadian cycles may be longer than twenty-four hours for sleep, body temperature, alertness, performance, and urinary electrolyte excretion. These tendencies may first appear during childhood. The internal circadian pacemaker in blind people may drive sleep and other biological functions so strongly that attempts to adjust the rhythms using time cues not related to light may not be successful.

You may recall that studies of sighted people showed that, in the absence of light cues, the human biological clock spans about 25.9 hours. (In chapter 4, we talked about how this was discovered through studies in which people stayed in bunkers without any cues of night and day). For sighted people, light cues reset this biological clock to coincide with the twenty-four-hour clock. Blind people's cycles are probably longer than twenty-four hours because they can't perceive the cues of light and dark that set the cycles for other people. Studies of their resulting sleep problems may help us solve the mystery of why some sighted people develop cycles longer than twenty-four hours, too.

How to Reset Your Body Clock

If you suffer from a sleep-phase disorder, you can use behavior modification techniques to resynchronize your internal circadian rhythm with the external world. These techniques can be quite challenging, but if you stick with the program carefully, they are quite effective.

Scheduling. Regardless of your sleep-phase disorder, one of the most important steps is to establish a regular schedule of bedtime and rise time. Set the schedule you want. Rely on your alarm clock and family to help rigorously enforce rise times and always adhere to your scheduled bedtime.

Chronotherapy. Chronotherapy is a brilliant way to help people with sleep-phase disorders realign their schedules. The strategy is that a person with delayed sleep phase syndrome goes to bed later and later each day until the bedtime cycles forward around the clock and reaches the designed bedtime. For example, if you were falling asleep regularly at three A.M. and rising regularly at eleven A.M., a chronotherapy schedule might require that you stay awake until six A.M. the first night and sleep no longer than two P.M.; on the second night, be awake until nine A.M. and sleep no later than five P.M.; on the third night, stay awake until noon and sleep no later than eight P.M.; and so on until you reach an appropriate nighttime bedtime and appropriate morning rise time. You then maintain that constant schedule to help lock in the new sleep/wake rhythm.

For advanced phase syndrome, where the problem is falling asleep earlier and rising earlier than desired, the goal again is to delay bed-times and rise times. However, the bedtimes are usually delayed by only a few hours. For example, if you routinely fall asleep at seven P.M. and rise at three A.M., the chronotherapy protocol might require you to remain active and alert every night until ten or eleven P.M. (the de-sired bedtime) to help shift the bedtime and rise time forward. This schedule would be maintained for several weeks to lock in the new sleep/ wake rhythm.

Bright Light. Circadian rhythm problems can also be treated by a pro-gram of exposure to bright light. You can expose yourself to natural sunlight at the appropriate time of day or a light box. For instructions on using a light box, see the section "Using Light to Alter Your Sleep Patterns" in chapter 4.

For delayed sleep phase syndrome, to reset the rhythm so sleep begins earlier, expose yourself to five thousand to ten thousand lux of light for thirty minutes or longer between six and nine o'clock in the morning. Avoid bright sunlight in the late afternoon and evening. You can get that much light from natural sunlight; ten thousand lux is bright sun at noon on a clear day. For advanced sleep phase syndrome, ex-pose yourself to the bright light in the late afternoon or early evening and avoid bright light in the morning. If you have used scheduling or chronotherapy to set a new rhythm for yourself, bright light can help lock in your new schedule.

Habits and Routines. After you have reset your sleep schedule, change your work, recreation, socialization, and meal times to fit it. For ex-ample, if you suffer from delayed sleep phase syndrome and routinely eat dinner at midnight, surf the Internet until 2:00 A.M., and then talk to your West Coast friends until 3:00 A.M., you should eat dinner earlier and enjoy your computer time and phone conversations earlier, making sure that all activities end before your scheduled bedtime. If you suffer from advanced sleep phase syndrome and rise early to drink coffee and catch the morning news, shift your schedule so that you watch the news in the evening and don't drink any coffee until after your scheduled rise time in the morning.

Two Examples. Maria, a university student, was worried because no matter what she did, she could not fall asleep until three A.M. and could not manage to get out of bed until noon. For years this sleep schedule had interfered with her class schedule, but she had managed to work around it. In a few months, though, she would graduate, and did not see how she could possibly hold down a job if she could not get to work before one in the afternoon!

After taking a careful history, completing sleep logs, and seeing Maria in the sleep laboratory, we determined that she suffered from delayed sleep phase syndrome. I recommended that she go to bed three hours later and rise three hours later on each successive night. On the first night she was to go to bed at six A.M. and rise at three P.M. On the next night she was to go to bed at nine A.M. and rise at six P.M. The next night she was to go to bed at noon and rise at nine P.M. It took about a week to advance her schedule around the clock so that she was going to bed at 11:00 P.M. and rising at eight A.M. Once she arrived at this desired sleep schedule, we asked her roommate to make sure Maria was up on time every morning. Maria also changed her habits of eating, studying, shopping, even telephoning. I also recommended exposure to bright light in the early morning just after awakening. Since it was winter, Maria used a bright light unit that she placed on a desk in her bedroom. Within weeks of making these behavioral changes and using the light therapy, Maria had achieved the schedule of nighttime sleep and daytime wakefulness that she wanted. And when she went out to interview for work, she landed the job that she wanted.

While Maria's problem was delayed sleep phase syndrome, Betty Jean had the opposite problem. A retired secretary in her mid sixties, she came to the sleep center because she thought she had insomnia. She said she fell asleep without any difficulty, slept for several hours, then awakened at 3:30 or 4:00 A.M. feeling "bright eyed and bushy tailed." She would often get up, make tea, have a bite of breakfast, and then spend several hours sitting in her house wondering what to do and feeling very lonely.

Since early-morning awakenings can sometimes be a sign of depression, I asked her whether she'd been feeling blue. She did not have the common signs of depression, and had no medical history of it. I then looked at her sleep log and talked to her about her sleep habits. Betty Jean began preparing for bed at around seven P.M. and would usually get into bed no later than eight P.M. She slept comfortably throughout the night until 3:30 or four A.M. This was not insomnia, but advanced sleep phase disorder.

Her treatment was simple and straightforward. Since she was getting about 7.5 or eight hours of sleep a night and wanted to rise between 7:30 and 8:00 A.M., I recommended that Betty Jean establish a bedtime of midnight. At first, she was perplexed by how to spend her evening hours, but she found it a much better time for socializing, pursuing hobbies, and even attending an occasional bingo game. When she was alone with her husband in the evenings, the two spent their

★☾★☾★☾★☾★☾★☾★

The Jury Is Still Out on Melatonin

Some studies have suggested that the hormone melatonin may help with sleep-phase disorders, but most sleep specialists are still quite cautious about recommending it as a sleep aid (see chapter 7).

Two studies have found that melatonin helped treat delayed sleep phase syndrome by encouraging earlier sleep onset. The hormone was given several hours before the usual time of sleep onset. No one has yet studied the use of melatonin to treat advanced sleep phase syndrome.

Some people have also suggested that melatonin may help treat jet lag. One large study of 474 people who took melatonin reported that they experienced fewer symptoms of jet lag. And at least one study has found that melatonin may speed one's recovery from jet lag when in the destination time zone. So, melatonin may be an effective aid in treating jet lag. More research is still needed.

time reading, playing board games, and watching new videos. In order to help Betty Jean delay her sleep onset, I also recommended bright light exposure in the late afternoon or early evening. She accomplished this by using a commercially available light box.

After only several weeks of treatment, Betty Jean was able to shift her sleep schedule. By staying awake later at night, she was able to remain asleep later into the morning. Staying awake later at night also allowed Betty Jean to spend more time with her husband, more time with her friends, and more time enjoying recreational pursuits.

✳ 9 ✳

Good Nights for Your Baby, Child, or Teen

If you are a parent, your sleep deprivation may have a straightforward cause: nighttime feedings, childhood nightmares, or staying up to make sure your teen gets home okay. Children have their own set of sleep problems. For their sake, and for yours, here are some insights into the differences between the ways children sleep and adults sleep and some practical solutions for common sleep problems.

SLEEPING LIKE A BABY

"Sleeping like a baby" refers to the way an infant drops effortlessly and naturally into sound, peaceful, restful sleep. In fact, sleep is one of the things newborns do best. Between meals, they sleep more than sixteen hours, or two-thirds of each day.

The sound, abundant sleep of a newborn doesn't have the distinct stages of sleep that an older child's and adult's has. An EEG won't show the same well-defined wave patterns of electrical activity in the brain. A full-term infant has two stages of sleep. About half of the time is spent in quiet sleep, characterized by closed eyes, sustained muscle tone, and breathing no more than twenty-five times a minute. The other half of the time is active sleep, with at least one eye movement, presence of twitches and brief head movements, and breathing more than twenty-five times a minute. Active sleep corresponds to REM sleep in adults. One has to wonder what kinds of images our little ones carry from their wakeful times into all those dreams. Many investigators have wondered why REM sleep occurs in such abundance in newborns. Years of research have suggested that this period is important for brain development. While the functions of REM sleep are still not fully known, we know that in lower animals REM sleep after birth is necessary for normal growth of brain cells.

As Dr. Spock and all parents know, definite patterns of sleep and wakefulness emerge and change as babies grow. Between the ages of one and three months, the pattern is polyphasic (poly = many, phasic = phases, polyphasic = "But I just put you down! You can't be ready to get up and be fed again!"). The rhythms of wakefulness and sleep can be as short as twenty minutes and as long as six hours. Long periods of wakefulness are usually followed by feeding, which is followed by long periods of sleep, in an ongoing cycle around the clock. The average duration of this cycle is approximately four hours, so a newborn may have five or six cycles of waking and sleeping in one day. This four-hour cycle may exist for several reasons, including the infant's immature nervous system and need to be fed at frequent intervals. All of which occurs, of course, on an entirely different rhythm than that of the parents! By the way, no difference occurs in nighttime awakenings between breast- and bottle-fed infants.

While these nighttime feedings are at first essential for an infant, supporting this pattern for too long can actually perpetuate awakenings beyond the point that Mother Nature intended. Weaning the baby from nighttime feedings is not just for mom and dad's convenience—it helps consolidate nighttime sleep into one uninterrupted stretch—and *consolidation of sleep is important for sleep development.* By about three months, babies who are fed during awakenings are less than half as likely to sleep through the night as those who are not fed during the night. By six months, most infants can forego nighttime feedings without experiencing hunger during the sleep period. Repeated feedings may condition the infant to awaken and demand food, creating an ongoing cycle of nighttime disruption.

During the first few months of life, the total amount of daily sleep time decreases from sixteen hours to fourteen or fifteen hours. By the age of eight months, this time is further reduced to thirteen or four-

✶☾✶☾✶☾✶☾✶☾✶☾✶

Colic and Sleep

A baby with colic cries loudly and for long periods when there is no apparent cause, such as hunger. Fortunately, colic almost always disappears by the third or fourth month. In the meantime, it is very disruptive not only to the parent's peace but also to the baby's sleep. A baby with colic can awaken frequently during the night and may take only sporadic, brief naps.

No specific treatment exists for colic, but it sometimes helps if the baby sleeps in a very quiet room and is handled gently. If you are breast-feeding, eliminating foods from your diet that can cause discomfort, such as milk or spicy foods, may help. If you are bottle-feeding, a change to soy formula may help. Talk to your pediatrician about steps you should take. Despite the extra difficulty, try to help your baby develop good sleep habits.

teen hours per day. By age two, sleep occupies only about twelve of every twenty-four hours. Over the first two years, REM sleep declines from one-half to one-third of the sleep period.

By the age of four or five months, the longest sleep period of the day is likely to occur at night. An association between the longest period of wakefulness and the longest period of sleep also develops; that is, a long period of wakefulness during the day is followed in the evening by the onset of the longest period of sleep.

As many as one-third of infants still awaken during the night by the end of their first year. Awakenings that persist after the first birthday may disappear as the child matures or may represent a sleep problem that is troubling to parents or other caretakers.

There is controversy about whether it's safest for a baby to sleep on his back, side, or face down. Each position poses some risk. On his back, the infant may aspirate fluids or vomit during sleep. On his tummy, he may lay face down into the bed. The tummy position has been associated with a higher risk of SIDs, sudden infant death syndrome. Currently the American Academy of Pediatrics recommends that parents place an infant on its back. Of course, once the baby can turn over, he will rearrange himself however he likes, but the risk of SIDs is lower by that age.

FROM *GOOD NIGHT, MOON* TO *THE BABYSITTERS CLUB*

Between the ages of two and five, total sleep time continues to decline slowly, the main sleep period of the day becomes more firmly positioned in the nighttime hours, and daytime sleep needs are satisfied by brief naps. During this period the child often establishes a daily routine that includes an afternoon nap, usually following lunch. My own son always waited until finishing his noon meal before napping. He intuitively knew that if he fell asleep before eating he would probably be awakened by hunger. As with most children, his after-lunch nap might last between one and three hours, and the refreshing effects of sleep were always evident in his renewed activity and demeanor.

While the sleep schedule is changing on the outside, exciting changes are also taking place in the brain's activity during sleep. The brain matures so that the full spectrum of brain electrical activity is represented during sleep. By the time the child reaches five years of age, an EEG will show all stages of sleep that an adult has. One of the most remarkable qualities of sleep during this period is the intensity of the deepest stages of sleep. Most young children *begin* the sleep period with a rapid descent into delta sleep, the deep sleep that adults reach only later. During such periods of delta sleep, the child may be extremely difficult to awaken and may not even be awakened by a full bladder or a noise or alarm that would wake up an older person. The intensity of delta sleep may be important to growth, since growth hormones are released during this stage. It may also be important for mental development.

Between the ages of six and eleven, sleep needs gradually fall. A six year old needs about nine hours of sleep, and a nine year old needs about eight and a half hours.

Encouraging Good Sleep Habits

Start as early as possible to help your child develop habits that promote good sleep and continue to encourage good habits throughout childhood. Your child will not only sleep better now but also learn how to develop good sleep habits on his own, a wonderful ability to take into adulthood.

Develop a Bedtime Routine. As early as possible, introduce a series of relaxing activities that you follow each night. Choose elements that are comfortable and enjoyable for both you and your child. Avoid rocking or patting the child to sleep, since the child will become overdependent on you over time. In one family, the routine includes a bath, a snack, toothbrushing, three picture books read in the child's bed, and then hugs and kisses. Your routine might include telling a story, reading the same book each night, singing a song, or choosing a stuffed animal companion. Over the years, the ritual will change along with your child. A child of ten might have the routine of getting into his pajamas, brushing his teeth, and reading for a short while before lights out.

Nap Routines Are Important, Too. Some children can nap anywhere they choose. Others need the security of a familiar place like their bedroom or car seat. Be sensitive to your child's need. Also, encourage napping at about the same time each day. This regularity helps you and your child anticipate periods of rest and activity and will help keep the child's sleep cycle regular.

Your Child's Sleep Environment. Just like adults, children need a comfortable place conducive to sleep. Keep your child's room dark, quiet, and at a comfortable temperature.

Comfort Objects. Toddlers and children can benefit from taking a special blanket or plush toy with them to bed. Offer your child several such objects and then include the chosen one in your bedtime ritual every night. For example, if he chooses a stuffed animal, he can snuggle with it while you tell a bedtime story and can keep it with him while he sleeps. The child will then associate the object with sleep, and its presence will ease the transition.

Sleep Problems in Childhood

A remarkable number of children have experienced a sleep-related problem. While some of these problems may be just bumps on the road to normal development, others are definitely a sign of delayed maturation, medical or psychological problems, or social and family influences. Whatever the source, a sleep problem can trouble both the parents and the child and interfere with the child's ability to function during the day.

The most common sleep problem among children is difficulty falling asleep. Whether you're a parent, aunt or uncle, occasional babysitter, or thank-goodness-this-isn't-my-problem dinner guest, you can easily recognize the hallmarks of this sleep problem: dilly-dallying and resistance when asked to get ready for bed; outright refusal to go to bed; frequent requests to get out of bed (or appearances, like a stubborn ghost, in the doorway); requests for "just one more story" or "another glass of juice"; responding to every noise; fears that arise while lying awake in bed; and restless sleep at the beginning of the night. Such problems can go on night after night after night.

Another type of problem that can emerge is the overproduced bedtime ritual. Simple rituals like taking a favorite blanket to bed or cuddling with a special stuffed animal are soothing and help most children go to sleep. However, sometimes these behaviors become a problem, especially when the parent must participate with a long period of cuddling, patting or rubbing the child's back, or rocking. At the extreme, sleep rituals can include potentially dangerous movements such as body rocking or head banging.

Nighttime awakenings are another common problem among children. After falling asleep at the beginning of the night, the child may be disturbed by frequent or long awakenings. This is especially common in children between the ages of one and three years. As the child gets older, the likelihood of nighttime awakenings declines dramatically. Fewer than 5 percent of children between the ages of three and eight report awakening frequently. Knowing that the problem can be outgrown may be comforting, but if you're the parent caught in this situation, a child who repeatedly awakens during the night and asks for you, asks for help returning to sleep, or asks to join you in your bed can be exhausting. You'll probably feel both frustration and guilt; you can't bear the ongoing disruption of your own sleep, but don't want your child to suffer, either.

Fortunately, parents dealing with a child's nighttime sleep problem don't have to just live with the problem until the child is older. Parents can take steps, even during early childhood, to help the child fall asleep and stay asleep. One of the first things to do is examine the sleep problem and the factors that might be contributing to it.

Sometimes the problem is napping at an age when most children have outgrown this need. This brings to my mind Robbie, a delightful four-year-old boy, and his mom, a nurse, who came to see me because Robbie couldn't fall asleep at night. He would lie awake in bed for more than an hour, making frequent requests to get up and watch videos or read books with his mom. A review of Robbie's sleep habits revealed that he was being cared for during the day by his elderly grandmother, who typically put him down for a long three- to four-hour nap in the middle of the afternoon. These naps were meeting part of Robbie's daily sleep need and making it more difficult for him to fall asleep at night.

I worked with the family, especially Robbie's grandma, who had a hard time gaining perspective on the problem. She even commented, "I don't know why they're having so much trouble with him at night. He sleeps just fine for me in the day!" On careful assessment, it became clear that Robbie's grandma found it taxing to be his full-time caretaker, so the naps were her way of getting a much-needed break. But this routine wasn't the best for Robbie, who needed more stimulation and less sleep during the day. A change in the child care arrangements, which gave Grandma some time off, and the enforcement of a regular sleep schedule, normalized Robbie's sleep in less than a week.

If your child isn't getting a three- to four-hour nap during the day and is experiencing sleeping problems, you should look for other contributing causes.

- **Could it be a medical problem?** Colds, flu, fever, ear infections, gastroesophageal reflux (a sudden, very unpleasant spurt of stomach contents or acid up the esophagus and into the back of the throat), or exposure to toxic substances such as lead are among the many medical problems that can contribute to difficulty falling asleep and nighttime awakenings. If a medical problem is the source of the problem, treatment of the underlying cause will usually reduce sleeplessness. However, in some cases the sleep problem persists long after the medical problem has resolved. In these cases, the parent should look for factors that may be perpetuating the sleep-lessness.

- **What about nighttime feedings?** As explained earlier, giving a bottle or other nutrition can contribute to nighttime awakenings. Elimination of feedings during the night can help the child consolidate sleep.

- **Are you sharing a bed?** Some researchers have found that children who sleep in the same bed with a parent are more likely to awaken during the night. If your child is sleeping with you and has sleep problems, you should examine what purpose this practice is serving and whether it should continue. Insisting that the child sleep in his or her own room can be challenging for the first few nights, but most children adapt quickly to sleeping alone. In the child who awakens frequently, this change may actually help consolidate sleep.

- **What kind of sleep habits have developed?** Some children develop poor sleep habits, sometimes with the unwitting collusion of their parents. Habits such as irregular bedtimes and rise times, irregular patterns of daytime activity and napping, eating a huge snack before bedtime, and failure to develop a bedtime routine can dramatically interfere with sleep onset or maintenance. In these cases, you need to identify the problem and then set firm limits to correct it.

- **What's your response to nighttime awakenings?** If your child awakens during the night, your natural response is to be concerned and attend to the child's needs. Depending on the nature of the awakening, though, you might wait a bit before entering the child's room, to see if the child will return to sleep on his own. Once in the room, try to keep the visit brief and boring. If you've already learned that your child will drift back to sleep without your intervention, avoid going into the room at all. Some parents immediately go to the child's side and initiate some action to help the child return to sleep. When repeated awakenings are met with repeated interventions, a cycle may develop in which the child is unable to return to sleep unless you intervene. This can actually promote more frequent or longer awakenings.

- **What is your child's transition to sleep like?** As described above, many children adopt a blanket or soft toy to help them get to sleep, and this crutch is fine. Small children like predictable routines, and good rituals are often very helpful. When transitions to sleep involve *you*, however, problems can develop. If you must be present to soothe, cuddle, pat, or rock the child, your own "adult" time in the evening (to say nothing of your patience) will suffer. The minute you stop patting and tiptoe to the door, the child will reawaken. In some situations, the child may awaken during the night, notice that you are gone, and insist that you return to help her get back to sleep. This behavior is a sure formula for long periods of wakefulness at the beginning of the night and frequent awakenings.

- **"Can I have just ten more minutes?"** The best approach is to be consistent about bedtimes. Children always test whether your rules really apply, again and again. If you allow your child to stay up late on some nights, and then refuse to allow it on other nights, your child will ply you for permission over and over again. If you waiver or give in, you may also give the impression that you are not in control, which can stir anxiety and distress just prior to bedtime. Setting firm and consistent limits helps to reinforce good sleep habits and assure your child that you are in control; therefore, all is well in the world, and it is safe to go to sleep.

- **Is fear a factor?** Many children have some fears at night. When these fears are intense and disrupt sleep, it's important for you to be as supportive as you can. While firm limits and remaining out of the bedroom may be good for other types of sleep problems, relax these rules when the child is truly suffering from fear at night. Showing the child that his fears are unfounded by exploring the room, checking the closet, looking under the bed, and experimenting with shadows can be a great comfort. You might put a bell at the child's bedside to "scare away ghosts" or to call for the immediate aid of a parent when fears become unbearable. In some cases, you may need to sleep in the same room with your child for a time.

- **Is the child experiencing psychological or social stress?** Children's sleep problems often occur in response to stress. Disputes between parents, separation, divorce, drug and alcohol problems, financial problems, and more can disrupt sleep. Even positive events—a vacation trip, a visiting relative—and relatively benign stresses, such as a change in routines at school, can give rise to a sleep problem. It is important to be sensitive to these factors and consider them when attempting to deal with your child's sleep difficulty.

Childhood Sleep Disorders

Studies have shown that 10 to 20 percent of children suffer from a sleep disorder like sleepwalking, tooth grinding, or bedwetting. Here are brief descriptions of sleep disorders that primarily affect children. For more about these conditions and their treatment, see chapter 10.

Sleepwalking. Common among young children, sleepwalking (somnambulism) peaks from nine to twelve years of age. The child may rise from bed and then go right back, or may move around the house or even outside. Throughout the episode, the child moves seemingly automatically, does not respond to the surroundings, and is difficult to arouse.

Nightmares. Almost every adult can recall having a nightmare as a child. Scary dreams that cause anxiety are common among children, particularly between the ages of seven and ten. However, very few parents say they worry about their children's nightmares or think treatment is necessary. A child awakened from a nightmare can usually recall a vivid, frightening dream. The child may be intensely afraid and may have difficulty returning to sleep. The best response is to give comfort and support. If frequent nightmares start to appear, seemingly out of nowhere, the child may be experiencing some stress.

Night Terrors. A child who has experienced a night terror awakens from sleep with intense fear and panic. The child may sit up in bed and begin screaming, but cannot describe a dream. In the morning, the child will have little or no memory of the event. While nightmares happen during REM sleep, night terrors happen during deep delta sleep. Also, children tend to react to a night terror more physically. Night terrors are most frequent between the ages of three and five, and they are usually rare events in the life of a child. Usually the problem resolves itself without treatment.

Confusional Arousals. The child awakens from sleep but is unresponsive. The parent may say the child "just seemed to look right through me."

Bedwetting. Wetting the bed during sleep is probably the most common childhood sleep problem. Most bed wetters are toddlers and preschoolers, but studies have shown that about 29 percent of children between the ages of four and fourteen had wet the bed recently. When the problem happens only once in a while, it is usually not treated. If it is frequent, a number of treatments are available (see chapter 10). It is important for you to be supportive of the child, who may be feeling distressed or guilty over the accident.

Sleep-Related Bruxism. Another sleep problem that affects children is tooth grinding or gnashing. The child does not realize that it is happening, but the parents may see or hear the grinding or the child may complain of a sore jaw or face in the morning. The child's dentist may see wearing down of the dental surfaces at a checkup. The best treatment is a dental appliance that protects the teeth.

Sleep Apnea. This disorder, uncommon in childhood, is a reduction or stopping of breathing for short periods during sleep. While it is normal for a child to have one or two episodes in which breathing is reduced during the night, the child with sleep apnea has several episodes a night. The condition fragments and disrupts sleep. In children, the cause can be enlarged tonsils or adenoids, and if so, removal can cause significant improvement. Sleep apnea can also be caused by structural problems in the face or head that interfere with the airway opening, such as a small and recessed jaw that might reduce the airway space behind the tongue.

TOO COOL TO SLEEP

Between twelve and twenty, young people need between eight and nine hours of sleep a night. However, while the youngest teens may spend about ten hours in bed at night, middle-adolescent children spend about eight and a half hours, and young adults of college age spend only about seven hours in bed per night. Many teens compensate for missed sleep during the week by sleeping very late on weekends. They may also fall asleep in classes or in front of the television—a sign that sleep deprivation is at work.

It seems likely, in fact, that older adolescents need even more sleep than preteens. Mary Carskadon, a professor at Brown University, tested the sleep patterns of young teens (pre- and early pubescent) and college students. The younger group was allowed to sleep up to ten hours a night, and the older group was allowed to sleep for seven or nine hours, their usual amount of sleep. Dr. Carskadon then gave both groups a multiple-sleep latency test, which offers opportunities to nap throughout the day. She found the younger kids were wide awake and alert all day, but the older kids were significantly sleepy all day long. On average, the younger kids took almost twenty minutes to fall asleep, which is normal, but the older kids fell asleep in less than five and a half minutes.

A message to get more sleep, especially in the first years of independence from established parental routines, may not be popular, but the stakes are high. Sleep deprivation is particularly likely among teens who have academic pressures, hold down a job, spend time with family, and socialize with friends. Often sleep deprivation leads to falling grades.

Lack of sleep takes on new urgency when your child becomes a driver. The teens are also a time when alcohol can become part of social situations for the first time. Not surprisingly, the combination of sleep deprivation and alcohol use is probably a significant cause of young drivers' high accident rates.

Like younger children, teens and young adults should follow good sleep habits and keep a regular schedule of bedtimes and rising times. A common cause of teenage sleep deprivation is trying to combine a job with the demands of homework and a social life. If the job is not economically essential, consider the wider impact that employment may have on your child's well-being. You may have to "just say no." Parents can try tying good sleep habits to certain rewards, but this approach is likely to motivate only younger teens. If your child is an athlete or values academic performance, it may help to talk about sleep as "powering up" for success.

Teens can experience any of the same sleep disorders that adults can, but such problems are rare at this age. Teens and young adults have outgrown the disorders common among younger children and are not old enough to have high rates of other disorders.

✲ 10 ✲

Sleep Disorders

In addition to insufficient sleep and insomnia, more than eighty other sleep disorders, each with distinctive signs and symptoms, can disturb nighttime sleep and disrupt daytime functioning. In this chapter, you'll learn how to recognize the most common sleep disorders so that if one affects you or someone you love, you can seek the proper treatment.

Frequently, people with a sleep disorder are able to sleep long enough each night, but their sleep is interrupted, fragmented, or disrupted. The result is sleep deprivation. A sleep disorder can also have other serious consequences. For example, a person with narcolepsy suffers from "sleep attacks," sleep paralysis, and other miseries. The nighttime activity associated with sleepwalking or REM sleep behavior disorder can lead to injury. Most of the disorders discussed in this chapter have significant physical or psychological effects.

SLEEP-RELATED BREATHING DISORDERS

Sleep-related breathing disorders include snoring, sleep apnea, and other conditions.

Snoring

A famous Italian actress, not especially known for her prowess as a nanny, volunteered to care for her friends' one-year-old baby. The parents were dubious, but off they went. When they arrived back home, they found the baby sitting on the floor, watching the sitter, who was sprawled on the sofa and snoring loudly. The actress opened one eye and said, "If I stop snoring for an instant, she yells." Apparently, the usual babysitting antics had failed to entertain the little one, but snoring did the trick.

That baby may be the only human in history to love listening to snoring. Kicking one's spouse—or kicking one's spouse *out*—for snoring probably began around the same time humans learned to walk upright.

Snoring is an audible, often *loud*, recurrent sound that occurs when a sleeper breaths in. Its volume and frequency vary. The sound is produced by the vibration of soft tissues in the airway, including the tonsils, soft palate, and uvula. Snoring happens when something—a small or narrow airway, nasal polyps, deviated septum—increases pressure in the airway when the person breathes in. The pressure pulls on the tissues of the upper airway until they vibrate. Snoring happens at night, but not during the day, because sleep decreases the tone of the muscles in the upper airway. Researchers believe that some snorers' airways actually collapse instead of opening when they breathe in, so the sleeper struggles noisily to inhale.

There are many among us who snore. In one survey of 5,713 adults, about 19 percent described themselves as habitual snorers (24.1 percent of the men and 13.8 percent of the women). The likelihood of snoring goes up with age. Up to thirty years of age, approximately 10 percent of men and less than 5 percent of women are habitual snorers. By age sixty to sixty-five, the incidence climbs to more than 60 percent of men and 40 percent of women.

Being overweight increases the chance that you will snore. Only 34 percent of people of healthy weight report habitual snoring, but more than 50 percent of people who are at least 15 percent above ideal weight say they snore. Hypothyroidism (low thyroid function) and tobacco are also linked with snoring. Snoring can suddenly and prominently increase because of nasal congestion from a cold or allergy, sleep deprivation, or the use of alcohol or sleeping pills.

Snoring never happens while you are awake, but it has an amazing capacity to begin as soon as you fall asleep. Snoring can also begin during the transition from wakefulness to sleep, at the first signs of Stage 1 sleep, or later in the sleep period. It can occur continuously or intermittently throughout the night and can happen during any of the sleep stages. Contrary to what might be expected, although breathing becomes less efficient during REM sleep, snoring appears to be softer and less frequent then than during the other stages. Snorers occasionally wake themselves up with their own noise, fragmenting sleep and leading to sleep deprivation.

Until recently, sleep specialists did not consider snoring a health problem, annoying as it can be. But new studies have suggested that snoring may be a symptom of a serious disorder. A large-scale study of habitual snorers have shown them at higher than usual risk of high blood pressure, heart disease, and stroke. It is not clear whether the increase is due to snoring or to sleep apnea of which snoring can be a sign. In fact, snoring is often the "wake up call" that brings someone with sleep apnea to the doctor in the first place. If you suffer from snoring and experience any symptoms of sleep apnea (see below), speak with your doctor about being seen at a sleep disorders center for evaluation and, if necessary, treatment.

Treatment. When it comes to snoring, desperation has been the mother of invention. Over the years, treatments have ranged from worthless tactics to devices worthy of medieval torture chambers, but there have been a few useful discoveries. One is that rolling over the snorer from the back to the stomach or side actually works. If your snoring is worse when you're sleeping on your back, try sleeping on your side.

Here are some other practical steps you can take to minimize or stop your snoring.

- Since snoring is worsened by being overweight, weight loss is often one of the best ways to reduce or eliminate it.
- Avoid alcohol, sleeping pills, and sleep deprivation, which all make snoring worse.
- If your snoring is associated with allergies or nasal congestion, use an air purifier for your room and a mild saline spray for your nose.

Avoid decongestant sprays, which can perpetuate, rather than cure, nasal stuffiness.

- One way to ensure that you'll sleep on your side is to sew a pocket in the middle of the back of an old T-shirt and put a tennis ball in it. Make sure that the ball fits tightly in the pocket so it doesn't roll around. Then wear the T-shirt to bed. When you roll onto your back, the tennis ball will be a gentle reminder to roll over.
- If your nasal passages are small or sometimes congested, you might try Breathe Rite nose tapes, which are available in drugstores.
- If your snoring is severe, your doctor may recommend that you see a dentist who can fit you with a device that minimizes snoring by keeping your jaw and tongue in place. You may also be a candidate for uvulopalatopharyngoplasty (UPPP) or laser-assisted uvulopalatoplasty (LAUP), surgeries that remove or reduce airway tissues.
- Be kind to your bed partner. Offer a comfortable set of ear plugs, just in case.

For Paul, as for many people, weight loss has helped reduce snoring. In his early thirties, Paul came to me because his snoring had become so loud it was annoying his wife. An overnight sleep test to rule out sleep apnea showed that Paul snored loudly in all body positions, so changing his sleep position would not help. Since the snoring had worsened over the past three years, and Paul had gained about twenty-five pounds during that time, I believed that shedding those extra pounds would improve the snoring significantly. Paul entered a weight-loss program to work toward that long-term solution, but he wanted to get rid of the snoring right away, so we recommended a dental appliance to keep his lower jaw forward and open up his airway. While the appliance didn't eliminate his snoring, it helped significantly. As Paul's weight dropped over the following months, he no longer needed the dental appliance. Weight loss did dramatically reduce his snoring.

Sleep Apnea

Sleep apnea is multiple interruptions of breathing during sleep. Breathing actually stops. The average pause lasts between thirty and forty seconds, but some have been timed at three minutes.

People with sleep apnea often also have events called hypopneas that partially reduce airflow. Though they are less complete than an apneic event, the oxygen in the blood declines and the hypopnea arouses the brain and muscles, causing a shift to a lighter stage of sleep.

The symptoms of sleep apnea include awakening gasping or choking; awakening for uncertain reasons, often with a sense of anxiety; restless sleep; unrefreshing sleep; morning headache; morning confusion; mood disturbance, including irritability and restlessness; and in men, inability to have an erection. Often, people don't acknowledge these symptoms ("There's nothing wrong with me, I'm just tired"), minimize the impact that the symptoms have on their lives, or attribute them to causes other than sleep disturbance.

One man who came to see me felt down in the dumps, lacked energy, was unable to enjoy the things he normally enjoyed, and was not doing well at work. Because it was winter, and he'd had similar problems during other winters, I thought he had seasonal affective disorder (SAD), a condition in which the natural decrease in light during fall and winter causes depression. Though the diagnosis was logical, given the symptoms, it was wrong, and the antidepressant medication prescribed for him failed to work. We then did sleep laboratory tests that revealed he had severe obstructive sleep apnea. The condition became worse during the winter because he gained weight then. The sleep apnea—not seasonal affective disorder—was the primary cause of his mood changes.

Sleep apnea affects between 1 percent and 10 percent of Americans. Recent data indicate that 2 percent of women and 4 percent of men between the ages of thirty and sixty years show some signs of sleep apnea syndrome. Sleep apnea may first appear at any age, but most cases are identified between the ages of forty and sixty. In women, it's more commonly diagnosed after menopause. The disorder increases with age. In studies of people over the age of sixty-five, investigators have found that 24 percent of people living independently, 33 percent in acute care inpatient facilities, and 42 percent in nursing homes have more than five apneic events per hour of sleep, the minimum amount required for a diagnosis of sleep apnea. Some have symptoms of the full syndrome and require treatment, and others don't.

Men and people who are obese are at greatest risk of sleep-related breathing disorders such as sleep apnea. Two-thirds of people with sleep apnea are obese. Excess upper body fat seems to be particularly linked to the condition. Some researchers recently found a high incidence of sleep apnea in Polynesian and South Pacific Island populations, possibly because of their inherited tendency toward obesity and excess fat in the upper body. Alcohol, central nervous system depressant drugs (such as the benzodiazepines), and sleeping on your back can also contribute to sleep apnea.

The only way to diagnose sleep apnea is an overnight evaluation in a sleep lab. A person is considered to have sleep apnea if he or she has at least five apneic or hypopneic events an hour, and at least forty events over eight hours. However, most people with sleep apnea have many more events. The average number of events per hour of non-REM sleep is seventy-nine, and the average number of events per hour of REM sleep is ninety. And some individuals have more than the average! As you can imagine, good sleep is impossible under these circumstances. The sleep is so fragmented that the amount of REM and delta sleep falls. The greater the degree of sleep fragmentation, the greater the daytime sleepiness. Apneic events also reduce the oxygen level in the blood, which can impair memory and motor skills the next day. The brain needs that oxygen.

The two most common signs of sleep apnea are snoring and excessive daytime sleepiness. Virtually all people with obstructive sleep apnea snore, and 94 percent of them say that they began snoring loudly before age twenty-one. Snoring in a person with sleep apnea is frequently loud and is interrupted by snorts or other unusual respiratory sounds. It's commonly a source of annoyance or embarrassment and can be very disturbing to a bed partner. Many individuals with sleep apnea have been evicted from their bedrooms because of loud snoring. Some report snoring so loudly that they have disturbed people in adjoining rooms or apartments.

People with sleep apnea usually complain of daytime sleepiness. Sleep laboratory tests have shown that people with sleep apnea fall asleep very quickly, averaging just 2.6 minutes to reach Stage 1 sleep during daytime naps. This means that they will have difficulty staying alert in many, many situations, perhaps even falling asleep at work, while socializing, at meal times, or driving. Be aware that you are at risk of an accident or injury when you experience such severe sleepiness. Note that for some folks, the only evidence of daytime sleepiness is fatigue or the tendency to doze at their desks or in other sedentary situations. If you snore at night, and are at all sleepy during the day, you should take these symptoms seriously.

Almost half of people with sleep apnea have irregular heartbeats, called cardiac arrhythmia. The heartbeat may become abnormally slow during an apnea event, then abnormally fast during respiration. If the blood oxygen levels fall low enough during the night, seizures can occur. An irregular heartbeat can be benign, serious, or life threatening. It is a sign that cardiac functioning is impaired.

People with sleep apnea have higher rates of high blood pressure and stroke. Also, they have higher death rates; the reason is not known, but it is believed that in many cases cardiopulmonary factors contribute to death. Because of related health risks, if you feel that sleep apnea may be an underlying cause of your sleep problems, see your doctor promptly; *then* try the other recommendations in this book if your doctor approves.

Treatment. If you have sleep apnea and you are obese, your doctor will probably tell you that you have to lose weight. Several studies have shown that for overweight individuals, losing weight through a diet can significantly reduce sleep apnea. Sometimes, even a slight decline in body weight (5 percent to 10 percent of total weight) can improve symptoms. However, as many of us know, weight loss is difficult to achieve and even more difficult to maintain. Because sleep apnea is a serious health problem, losing weight is *important* for you. If you are having trouble losing weight, talk to your doctor about structured weight-loss programs, medications, and surgical procedures. You need to choose an approach that can keep the weight off over the long run, since your symptoms will return if you gain the pounds back.

A highly effective, common treatment for sleep apnea is called "nasal continuous positive airway pressure." A mechanical device delivers room air to the nasal airway through a mask at a pressure that is sufficient to keep the upper airway open. This treatment significantly reduces the number of apneic and hypopnetic events and may even eliminate them. In initial nights of therapy, delta and REM sleep rebound. Long term, daytime sleepiness and blood pressure improve, as do mental performance and psychological well-being. The machine must be used nightly. Most studies have found that long-term home use is safe and effective. Major complications are rare. The greatest limiting factor in continued treatment is that, for various reasons, some people don't stay with it. It helps when people continue to follow up with their doctors during treatment.

Nasal continuous positive airway pressure made a huge difference for Ed, a middle-aged technical writer who first sought treatment because he was falling asleep in front of his computer monitor. When I talked to Ed, he reported several symptoms of sleep apnea: loud snoring, restless sleep, morning headaches, and fatigue throughout the day. He was taking medication for high blood pressure. An overnight laboratory test confirmed that he had severe sleep apnea—he totally stopped breathing more than sixty times per hour, and partially stopped breathing more than thirty times per hour.

We brought Ed back to the laboratory so that we could start treatment with nasal continuous positive airway pressure. He slept overnight again so that we could adjust the machine. Once we achieved the right pressure, Ed's breathing became regular and his oxygen levels remained normal throughout the night. Also, he got the delta and REM sleep he'd been missing. He awakened that morning feeling refreshed and bright, claiming, "I haven't slept this well in years." We arranged to have a machine sent to Ed's home, where he has been using it nightly for several months. He is no longer suffering from daytime sleepiness. We have also heard from Ed's family doctor that he no longer needs as much medication for his blood pressure.

Another treatment is a tongue retainer that opens the airway by moving the tongue and lower jaw forward. This device can significantly reduce apneic events in some people. It is most likely to help if the person has mild apnea, and apnea while lying on the back, but not stomach or side. Other in-the-mouth appliances have had some, but still limited, success.

In some cases, sleep apnea can be treated surgically. Uvulopalatopharyngoplasty is a procedure that enlarges the airspace in the back of the throat by shortening the uvula and soft palate. This surgery improves sleep apnea about half the time, but may not totally eliminate it. Success rates have been reported to be higher when evaluations before the operation include careful evaluation of the airway. Possible complications include postoperative bleeding and severe sore

✴☾✴☾✴☾✴☾✴☾✴☾✴☾✴

If You Think You Have Sleep Apnea

- Sleep apnea is a serious disorder that requires medical attention. See your doctor.
- Pursue evaluation and treatment at a sleep center!
- Try to lose weight, but don't rely on weight loss as the only treatment.
- Alcohol, sleeping pills, and sleep deprivation can worsen sleep apnea, so avoid them all.
- If you have allergies or nasal congestion, use a room air purifier and a mild saline nasal spray. Avoid decongestant sprays.
- If you're sleepy during the day, don't place yourself or others at risk by driving or operating machinery.
- Snoring may be the only warning mechanism that alerts you to sleep apnea. If you are treated for snoring, make sure you are checked for apnea, too,
- For more information regarding sleep apnea contact the American Sleep Apnea Association at 2025 Pennsylvania Avenue, N.W., Suite 905, Washington, DC, 20006, 202-293-3650. This organization can provide a brochure and other publications that describe sleep apnea and appropriate treatment options. The brochure includes a self-examination with a "snore score" that will tell you if your snoring could be a signal for sleep apnea.

throat, and, more rarely, long-term problems with nasal reflux (fluids washing up the back of the nose) and difficulty vocalizing certain sounds. A newer procedure called laser-assisted uvulopalatoplasty, which removes or reduces airway tissues with a laser, appears to be a poor treatment for apnea, though it can help with snoring.

If sleep apnea is linked to a nasal condition that interferes with airflow, such as polyps or a deviated septum, nasal reconstruction surgery may help.

Upper-Airway Resistance Syndrome

Another sleep-related breathing disorder, only recently identified, is upper-airway resistance syndrome, which moderately reduces airflow during sleep. These reductions often are not detected by conventional recording methods but can be diagnosed with an esophageal balloon test. Although the changes in respiration are subtle and may be as short as three seconds, they can cause arousals during sleep that are similar to those seen in sleep apnea. The primary symptom of upper-airway resistance syndrome is daytime sleepiness. The condition is treated the same way as sleep apnea.

People with sleep apnea may also have episodes of upper-airway resistance, although the two disorders are entirely separate.

Obesity Hypoventilation Syndrome

Obesity hypoventilation syndrome (Pickwickian syndrome) is often associated with sleep apnea, although it may be found alone. In this rare syndrome, less air than usual enters the air sacks of the lungs, leading to low levels of oxygen in the blood and retention of carbon dioxide that should be leaving the body. Unlike sleep apnea, which occurs in events, this syndrome affects the person all the time, night and day, but is more pronounced during sleep. It is caused by excessive weight on the lungs and respiratory muscles and worsens when the person lies on the back. Lung disease, upper-airway resistance, or diaphragmatic dysfunction adds to the mechanical load the struggling muscles must overcome. The condition can be life threatening.

Episodes of hypoventilation are often followed by arousals similar to those that follow apneic and hypopneic events. These arousals may prevent or disrupt deep sleep and may awaken the sleeper many times. Consequently, the symptoms may include disturbed nighttime sleep and excessive daytime sleepiness. However, some people are not aroused or awakened, even when very low levels of oxygen are reaching the tissues and carbon dioxide levels are excessively high, conditions that could harm the heart and lungs. Since they are not aroused, they may not report symptoms of disturbed sleep.

Treatment. Obesity hypoventilation syndrome is treated with supplemental oxygen to eliminate low oxygen levels. Diuretic medication (water pills) can reduce water retention and swelling in the lungs and the rest of the body. Reduction of upper-airway resistance can be critical. Treatment may include the use of nasal continuous positive airway pressure (see page 180), positive-pressure ventilation (using a machine that facilitates breathing mechanically), and nasopharyngeal or endotracheal intubation. When these measures fail, an opening in the windpipe, called a tracheostomy, may be made and secured with a plastic button. However, even this aggressive last resort may have disappointing results. Weight reduction is always recommended as a long-term treatment strategy in treating obese people with this disorder.

NARCOLEPSY

People with narcolepsy experience sudden and irresistible urges to sleep during the daytime. Such "sleep attacks" may last for a few minutes or even as long as an hour. Sometimes people with narcolepsy do something—even something quite complex—without later being aware that they did it. Sometimes the behaviors are quite disorganized and illogical.

Some people with narcolepsy experience *hypnogogic hallucinations*, visual or auditory experiences that occur just before sleep begins or just upon awakening. Visual experiences sometimes involve black-and-white or colored geometric shapes, but may also include more defined images of animals or people. Auditory experiences may include strange sounds or voices. In some cases, the individual may experience a tactile hallucination, perhaps feeling the touch of a hand on his shoulder.

Another sign of narcolepsy is *sleep paralysis*, brief periods when you can't move your muscles *while you are awake*. Having sleep paralysis doesn't mean that you suffer from narcolepsy, but the two often go together. Sleep paralysis provokes anxiety. It renders you unable to move your arms or legs, talk, or even open your eyes, and you have full memory of the event. As if this were not frightening enough, sleep paralysis sometimes occurs in conjunction with hypnogogic hallucinations. Imagine being unable to move while experiencing a frightening or threatening hallucination! One woman described being unable to move while experiencing a hypnogogic hallucination that someone was outside her door talking about killing her.

The last symptom that points to narcolepsy is *cataplexy*, sudden loss of muscle tone during wakefulness that is commonly brought on by a strong emotion such as laughter or anger. A cataplectic attack can be mild and involve only a few muscles, such as a sudden loss of muscle tone in the head and neck causing the head to droop. Or the attack can be severe, with complete loss of muscle tone, causing the individual to drop helplessly to the ground. While attacks are usually short, they can last as long as thirty minutes.

Narcolepsy is a disorder of REM sleep. We know this because people with narcolepsy enter a period of REM sleep when they fall asleep at night or in a nap. Hypnogogic hallucinations, sleep paralysis, and cataplexy may be manifestations of REM sleep that occur during wakefulness.

Narcolepsy is rare, affecting less than 1 percent of the general population, but it significantly affects the sufferer's quality of life and ability to function during the day. People with narcolepsy must also deal with others' reactions, which are often less than sympathetic. The disorder can affect friendships, family relationships, and work life.

Narcolepsy has a genetic component, as the condition tends to run in families. The symptoms usually first appear between the ages of fifteen and twenty-five but can appear earlier or later.

Treatment. If you think that you have narcolepsy, you should consult promptly with your doctor or a sleep specialist. Daytime sleepiness is usually controlled with stimulant medication, such as methylphenidate (Ritalin) or pemoline (Cylert). Antidepressants, such as the tricyclics protriptyline (Vivactyl) or imipramine (Tofranil), are usually added to control hypnogogic hallucinations, sleep paralysis, and most important, cataplexy. Some newer medications have been developed for narcolepsy, such as modafinil, which may soon be approved for use in the United States, and gamma hydroxybutyrate, which is currently available only in Europe and Canada.

While most people with narcolepsy initially pursue treatment with medication, it's not an easy route. The relief provided by medications ranges from minimal to maximal, and some of the medications used may cause adverse reactions. Open communications with your health care provider are a key element of successful treatment of narcolepsy.

Some people with narcolepsy can successfully manage daytime sleepiness with periodic naps. Some find that their symptoms worsen after they eat; dietary strategies, such as decreasing food intake or avoiding specific foods, may help manage their symptoms.

Treatment is often multifaceted, as it is for Ermine, a receptionist in her early twenties who has narcolepsy. She takes a low dose of stimulant medication to help her stay awake during the day and a low dose of tricyclic medication to relieve the symptoms of cataplexy. She also uses naps to improve her daytime alertness. Finally, Ermine has had individual and family therapy so that she and her loved ones can learn to accept the nature of her illness and deal with some of the struggles that face them. While Ermine's symptoms have not been totally relieved, she says they are only a fraction as bothersome as they were before she began treatment.

If you would like more information on narcolepsy, contact the Narcolepsy Network at P.O. Box 1365, FDR Station, New York, New York 10150. This group offers an excellent support network as well as information regarding the illness.

SLEEP-RELATED MOVEMENT DISORDERS

Movement disorders cause part of the body to move during sleep, resulting in arousal and fragmentation of sleep.

Restless Legs Syndrome

Restless legs syndrome is tingly, "creepy crawly" feelings in the limbs that cause the person to move (sometimes vigorously), stretch, massage the legs, or get out of bed and walk, to gain relief. It occurs *just prior to sleep onset or during awakenings that occur during the sleep period.* The movements can be minor, even unnoticeable, perhaps flexing the muscles of the foot, or they can be forceful twitches or kicks that startle the sleeper. The level of movement varies from person to person and even from night to night. In severe cases, movements may be present during relaxed daytime wakefulness, which can be both uncomfortable and annoying. When the discomfort persists and the movements continue, the sleeper can feel helpless and become agitated, angry, or even depressed.

The leg movements typical of this syndrome can significantly delay the start of sleep. They commonly occur while the sleeper is passing from wakefulness to Stage 1 sleep, making it difficult to gain the momentum that is needed to enter deeper stages of sleep. The overall impression is of insomnia or unrefreshing sleep.

Certain factors can contribute to the appearance or worsening of restless legs syndrome. It is more common among older people. The syndrome may have a genetic component, as more than half of people with the disorder have at least one family member who is also affected. The use of caffeine or nicotine, especially in the late afternoon or evening, may make the syndrome worse. Other contributing factors can include certain drugs (especially some antidepressant medications), withdrawal from certain drugs (including sedative hypnotics), pregnancy, strenuous exercise, peripheral neuropathy, diabetes, anemia, and some other medical conditions.

While some cases can be identified on the basis of their symptoms, diagnosis typically requires overnight testing in a sleep laboratory (see chapter 11). Treatment is identical to that for periodic limb movement disorder, which is described below.

For more information contact the Restless Legs Syndrome Foundation at 304 Glenwood Avenue, Raleigh, North Carolina, 27603-1455. This group publishes a newsletter that is available to the public.

Periodic Limb Movement Disorder

Periodic limb movement disorder causes leg movement, and possibly arm movement, during sleep. The movements are brief, typically lasting between half a second and five seconds. While the movements can take place at any point during the sleep period, they tend to be worst at the beginning of the night. They are typically present during Stages 1 and 2 of sleep, and less so during delta and REM sleep. The movements also tend to occur in runs or series with one movement taking place at least every twenty to forty seconds for several minutes during the sleep period. The movements can occur in the left leg alone, the right leg alone, or in both legs at once. In some cases the legs move alternately as if pedaling a bike.

As in restless legs syndrome, the movements range from slight muscle flexes to big movements of the legs or arms that can jolt the sleeper or bed partner right out of bed. Unquestionably, these movements, even the slight ones, disrupt sleep. Movements commonly bring the sleeper's brain into a state of wakefulness for a few moments. After such an arousal, the sleeper typically drifts back into Stage 1 sleep, and may even reach deeper stages. However, the next movement that occurs—usually in less than a minute—creates another arousal and sleep stage change, creating cycles of sleep disruption. Although the sleeper is usually not aware of the dozens or even hundreds of awakenings, some may be perceived or prolonged, so it's common for a person with periodic limb movement disorder to have insomnia. If the sleeper does not wake up during the events, he may just describe his sleep as nonrestorative or unrefreshing.

Periodic limb movement disorder becomes more common with age. The disorder has the same contributing factors as restless legs syndrome, including caffeine and nicotine use, muscle fatigue, and a variety of medical conditions.

Restless legs syndrome and periodic limb movement disorder can occur together. The person will experience one while lying awake in bed, and the other after falling asleep. This sequence suggests that both disorders may have the same cause, which is supported by the fact that the same medications can treat both dissorders.

One person who had both sleep disorders was an actress in her late fifties who came to the sleep center because unusual sensations in her legs were making it difficult for her to fall asleep. In an overnight laboratory test, electrodes on her legs revealed ever-so-slight muscle activity that aroused her every time she began to drift off to sleep. They also showed that the muscle twitches continued after she was asleep—more than 120 times an hour. All this movement elevated the amount of Stage 1 sleep and reduced the amount of deep sleep, resulting in sleep deprivation. Treatment with the medication Pergolide (Permax) dramatically improved her symptoms.

Treatment. An effective drug treatment for both restless legs syndrome and periodic limb movement disorder is Sinemet, which is a combination of the drugs L-dopa and carbidopa. This medication was initially developed for the treatment of Parkinson's disease. The dose is low at first and is raised until symptoms improve. A sustained release form of the medication can be taken if the regular form wears off before the night is over. The effectiveness of Sinemet has led researchers to evaluate similar medications. The ones used most successfully have been pergolide (Permax) and bromocriptine (Parlodel). Codeine may help, but it must be used with great caution, as it may be addictive.

For more information contact the Restless Legs Syndrome Foundation, Inc. at 304 Glenwood Avenue, Raleigh, North Carolina, 27603-1455.

Nocturnal Paroxysmal Dystonia

Nocturnal paroxysmal dystonia causes writhing and flailing motions during sleep. The episodes may last only a few seconds or as long as an hour. The movements can severely fragment sleep, making it unrefreshing. They can also lead to awakenings and complaints of insomnia. There's no evidence of epilepsy in people with nocturnal paroxysmal dystonia, and the relationship between these two disorders is unclear.

Treatment is sometimes successful using the medication carbamazepine (Tegretol). Treatment has also been tried with phenytoin (Dilantin) and barbiturate medications.

PARASOMNIAS

Parasomnias (the term means "around or about sleep") are abnormal behaviors during sleep, such as sleepwalking, bedwetting, nightmares, and other problems. These behaviors can lead to sleep deprivation by disrupting sleep or causing awakenings.

Sleep-Related Bruxism

Sleep-related bruxism is tooth grinding during sleep. The upper and lower jaws chew or gnash together for a few seconds at a time. Some people make slight movements that are barely noticeable, while others suffer from intense flexing of the jaw muscles and very loud tooth-grinding sounds. There are "war stories" told by people who have been awakened by the noise of a person with bruxism in the next room.

Bruxing usually occurs in episodes during the night. In severe cases, many episodes can occur during a single night of sleep. Sleep-related bruxism is a common problem among children and adolescents, but it can also affect adults. Studies have reported that between 5 and 20 percent of Americans have had the problem.

Bruxing occurs during all stages of sleep, but is most likely during Stage 2 sleep. It causes arousal from sleep; some episodes may even provoke an awakening, which can lead to the perception of insomnia or unrefreshing, nonrestorative sleep. However, most people who suffer from sleep-related bruxism are probably not aware that they are grinding their teeth at night. They are usually informed of the problem by a family member or bed partner or by pain in their jaw muscles upon awakening in the morning. Sleep-related bruxism is frequently first suspected by a dentist who notices worn dental surfaces.

The causes of sleep-related bruxism are unknown. However, it's known that sleep-related bruxism is more likely to occur during times of stress. It also seems to run in families, so you are more likely to suffer from bruxism if your parents or siblings have the problem. Finally, some relationship may exist between uneven dental surfaces (malocclusion) and the occurrence of sleep-related bruxism. Some experts have suggested that a tooth grinder may be trying to wear down such uneven surfaces.

Treatment. The most common treatment is a mouth guard worn during sleep. Fitted by a dentist, the device will not reduce bruxing activity, but does prevent damage or wear to dental surfaces. Psychotherapy, relaxation techniques, or biofeedback can reduce the stress and muscle tension that contribute to bruxing.

Sleep Talking

Talking in your sleep is a common phenomenon, particularly among children. The vocalizations range from simple sounds, such as a moan or grunt, to complex statements. Sleep talkers may express strong emotions like anger and may even become tearful.

It's a fallacy that sleep talkers are revealing their innermost secrets. For one thing, it would be next to impossible to sort out what's the secret and what's babbling. If you want to know someone's secrets, get some sleep and ask the person in the morning.

Another fallacy is that most sleep talkers talk during their dreams. Sleep talking occurs in non-REM sleep about 80 percent of the time. However, when talking does occur during REM sleep, it's quite likely to reflect the content of the dream. While sleep talking can result in arousal from sleep, this is rarely a problem, as it doesn't appear to significantly fragment sleep. Sleep talking rarely requires any treatment.

Sleepwalking

Sleepwalking is walking during sleep. It can take the form of sitting up in bed, wandering, or engaging in some activity. Sleepwalking oc-

★ ☾ ★ ☾ ★ ☾ ★ ☾ ★ ☾ ★ ☾ ★ ☾ ★

Protecting Yourself If You Sleepwalk

- *If you believe your sleepwalking occurs when you are under stress, try to reduce the sources of stress in your life.*
- *Avoid sleep deprivation and avoid alcohol, which worsen sleepwalking. Also be aware that medications you are taking may influence the frequency or severity of your sleepwalking.*
- *Protect yourself from injury by securing your sleep environment. For example, before you go to bed at night, make sure that sharp or glass objects are out of any path you might wander. Lock your windows and cover them with attractive, locking shutters or thick drapes. Lock your doors. Move your bedroom to the ground floor if you fear that you may stumble down the stairs while sleepwalking.*
- *Trying to arouse or awaken a sleepwalker can sometimes make things worse. She can be startled or frightened and respond by flailing about or striking out. It's best to gently guide the sleepwalker back to bed and encourage her to lie down.*

curs during delta sleep, so it often happens in the first two or three hours of sleep when the longest periods of deep sleep occur. Since it does not happen during the REM period, it is not the acting out of dreams. In the morning, the person has no memory of the sleepwalk.

Sleepwalking is most likely in childhood. Many children walk in their sleep at least once. You are ten times more likely to be a sleepwalker if your mother, father, or siblings are. While sleep-walking episodes may become more frequent during times of stress, especially in adults, there's no evidence that they are a sign of a psychiatric disorder.

Treatment. Sleepwalking is so common, and often seems so harmless, that most people don't report it at their health checkups. When sleepwalking occurs frequently, however, or if the sleepwalker puts himself at risk of injury, tell your doctor or pediatrician. For example, the sleepwalker may cut himself by rustling through a kitchen drawer full of sharp knives or may walk outside into the street while asleep.

In many cases, the doctor will recommend securing the sleep environment; in serious cases, medication can be used to reduce the number of episodes. Medications such as the benzodiazepines (see chapter 7) and tricyclic antidepressants have helped adult sleepwalkers, but these medications are not commonly given to children. If sleepwalking occurs only during times of stress, psychotherapy may be appropriate. Counseling, relaxation therapy, and even hypnosis have helped some sleepwalkers. Consider these options with your doctor.

Nocturnal Eating Syndrome

Nocturnal eating disorder is a pattern of eating during the sleep period, either consciously or as a form of sleepwalking. The person is unable to return to sleep without eating or drinking but afterwards goes to sleep without difficulty.

One type of nocturnal eating is a form of sleepwalking in which the person rises from bed, obtains food, and then returns to bed with little or no memory of the eating episode. If awakened, the person rarely reports hunger or thirst that might account for the compulsive and immediate urge to consume food at night. Eating behavior is often impulsive and sloppy. The person may eat normal foods like a sandwich or leftovers, or make bizarre choices like uncooked spaghetti or rice, raw bacon, cat food, or an entire jar of mayonnaise. Some night eaters will even try to consume nonfood items, such as a scouring pad or an oven mitt. The sleeper probably won't be aware of what has happened until the mess is surveyed in the morning.

Another kind of night eating has been observed in very obese people, those whose weight is posing a serious threat to their health. They are more likely to be aware of their night eating and report that they were hungry or thirsty but may be reluctant to acknowledge the severity of their binges. Often daytime dieting plays a role, with the fewer the calories consumed during the day, the more consumed at night.

Nocturnal eating syndrome has also been observed in people with the eating disorder bulimia, which during the day often involves eating large amounts and then purging the food through vomiting or laxatives. Binge eating may also occur at night. The person eats in a disorganized way while sleepwalking and does not remember the events upon awakening.

Nocturnal eating syndrome can cause daytime fatigue and sleepiness due to periods of wakefulness at night. It can also contribute significantly to calorie consumption and weight gain. In fact, studies suggest that failure to lose weight despite adherence to dietary restrictions during the day may sometimes be caused by this kind of food consumption during the sleep period.

Night eating may worsen sleep-related breathing disorders like sleep apnea or snoring by interfering with weight loss or adding to weight gain.

Treatment. Treatment with a benzodiazepine medication (see page 133) can help sustain sleep and reduce or eliminate eating during sleep.

Obese people who consume food during sleep may need to modify their weight-loss diet, slightly increasing daytime calories to avoid a rebound effect at night. Another suggestion is to prepare a tray of low-calorie food that can be consumed during nighttime awakenings. Finally, if the person has sleep apnea (obese people are at greater risk), treating that disorder may help sustain sleep and reduce the number of eating episodes. People with eating disorders such as bulimia need to seek treatment for the underlying disorder as well as the sleep problem.

REM Behavior Disorder

A person with REM disorder acts out his dreams because the mechanism that usually suppresses muscle activity during REM sleep is not functioning properly. A rare disorder, it affects mostly men over the age of sixty. Most cases are not associated with a significant medical or psychiatric illness.

For an unknown reason, the dreams of people with REM behavior disorder tend to be filled with action and violence. Consequently, the sufferer may act out a dream by yelling, screaming, punching, kicking, or attacking. Despite the vigorous activity that takes place during the night, these bedroom Chuck Norrises can awaken feeling refreshed and alert, although some describe their sleep as restless, fitful, or unrefreshing.

One austere, elderly gentleman who suffered from REM behavior disorder had worked as a hotel doorman for many years. He later devoted himself to charity work at his church. This man was nonviolent, had never had any interest in fighting, and had never taken a single martial arts class, but he came to my office at the insistence of his wife, who reported that he would nightly sit up in bed, begin yelling profanities, rise from bed, and then deliver karate punches and kicks to some imaginary enemy. If gently awakened, he could immediately recall a violent dream and could easily be guided back to bed. However, his wife had become increasingly reluctant to intervene, after getting flung to the floor and bruised by her kung fu husband! Both husband and wife were afraid that he would harm himself or his wife, so he followed through with a complete evaluation and treatment.

While sleepwalking arises from the delta sleep abundant at the beginning of the night, REM behavior disorder happens during REM sleep, which is more abundant late in the last third of the night. When abnormal behaviors occur later in the night, they are more likely to be REM related.

Treatment. If you think you may have REM behavior disorder, see your doctor for a general checkup to rule out other health problems, particularly neurological disorders such as a degenerative brain disease. You may have a CT scan or MRI. You should also be evaluated at an accredited sleep disorders center.

Some medications are highly effective in treating REM behavior disorder. Clonazepam (Klonopin) in low doses at bedtime is effective in nearly 90 percent of people with REM behavior disorder. Other benzodiazepine medications, as well as some tricyclic (antidepressant) medications, have also been used successfully.

Bedwetting

Bedwetting (sleep enuresis) is involuntary urination during sleep. One-third of four year olds, 10 percent of six year olds, and 5 percent of ten year olds wet their beds. The problem is more common among boys than girls. It is caused by a failure to respond to normal bladder signals during sleep.

Before the age of five, bedwetting is considered normal. When an older child continues to wet the bed, perhaps nightly or sometimes even several times per night, it can become a serious problem. The child may feel embarrassed and the parents may feel frustrated. Bedwetting can also be associated with sleepwalking or night terrors.

Bedwetting can also develop later, in adolescence or adulthood. The cause can be medical illness, bladder dysfunction, mental retardation, or severe psychiatric illness.

Treatment. The treatment depends on the severity of the problem, the child's age, and the concerns of the child and parents. If the child is three or four, the problem may be outgrown. The "big kid" disposable training pants on the market (less embarrassing than diapers) can be worn nightly until the problem eases. If the child is older or the problem more troubling for the family, here are some other treatment options.

- Bladder training, in which the child is given fluids during the day and then asked to delay urination for as long as he can, can train the bladder to hold more.
- Another type of bladder training for children challenges them to start and stop the stream of urine several times during urination. This may give the child a greater sense of control.
- Alarms can help train the sleeper to wake up when the need to urinate arises. A pad is placed under the sheets. When it becomes wet, it sounds the alarm.
- Both children and adults with bedwetting may be helped by medication. Low doses of tricyclic medications (antidepressants), taken at bedtime, may reduce the need to urinate.

If you are an older person who has problems with leaking urine during the night, see your doctor for diagnosis and treatment. Help is available—you don't need to just suffer in silence. See the section on urinary frequency on page 41.

Nightmares

Nightmares are dreams filled with fear and anxiety. They are quite common, occurring at least occasionally in about 75 percent of children and 50 percent of adults. Frequent nightmares, though, are quite rare.

Nightmares are prolonged dreams with frightening content that may be present at the beginning of the dream but more typically evolves as the dream progresses. Often the dream includes a threat of physical attack or injury. By definition, nightmares always arise from REM sleep. They are both vivid and convoluted. The nightmare is often but not always followed by an awakening during which the sleeper is often disturbed by the content of the dream. The person, especially a child, may be afraid to remain in bed or return to sleep.

Nightmares that occur in adults can be a sign of stress. Chronic stress can lead to extended periods of recurrent nightmares. For example, an individual going through a painful divorce might have several nights of disturbing dreams. Nightmares can also be a reaction to a past stress. They are one of the most troubling parts of post-traumatic stress disorder (see page 47) In some cases, the appearance of nightmares in an adult is a sign of a more serious psychiatric problem.

Some medications may increase the likelihood of nightmares, especially medications such as L-dopa and beta blockers (for example, propranolol). Also, withdrawal from REM sleep-suppressing drugs such as the tricyclics may give rise to nightmares.

Treatment. In children treatment of nightmares is rare, as they are considered common and unharmful. In adults, treatment must take into account the frequency and severity of the nightmares as well as their possible underlying cause. If the nightmares are significantly troubling, a thorough evaluation is necessary to rule out medical, psychiatric, and medication-related causes. In the absence of such problems, nightmares may be treated with psychotherapy, medication (such as the benzodiazepines or tricyclic antidepressants), or a combination of both.

Sleep Terrors

Sleep terrors are awakenings from delta sleep—not from REM sleep—during which the individual experiences intense fear that is believed to be related to some mental content that occurred just prior to the awakening, but which the sleeper cannot describe well. Sleep terrors are rare in young children and adults, and more common among older children and adolescents. Approximately 3 percent of children and 1 percent of adults have experienced a sleep terror.

A person experiencing a sleep terror typically screams loudly and then wakes fully, often agitated. Some children jump out of bed and wildly run about the room as if escaping something fearful. The child is very difficult to console and may strike out if a parent attempts to be soothing. The episode usually lasts only a few minutes after which the child is usually unable to describe what was so frightening. He may say "something was going to get me" or "monsters got me" but be unable to elaborate further.

When sleep terrors occur in adults, they may become more frequent or severe under stress.

Treatment. When sleep terrors are rare occurrences, they are usually not treated. However, when they are frequent, treatment may be called for. The most typical treatment for children is psychotherapy. Medications are available that may help, but these are usually taken only by adults.

Confusional Arousals

In a confusional arousal, the person, usually a toddler or preschooler, is jarred from deep delta sleep. Disoriented and confused, the child may move about in bed or cry. The child may be unresponsive or may act inappropriately. Some parents have described their child as "not recognizing me" or "looking right through me."

An episode may last several minutes or even longer than an hour. They always go away by themselves. In fact, efforts on the part of a parent to awaken or startle the child may even prolong the episode.

Rhythmic Movement Disorder

Rhythmic movement disorder is head banging, head rolling, body rocking, or other rhythmic movements during sleep. It affects only children. Many infants do these things to some extent, but the problem becomes less likely as the child grows older. The movements commonly occur for less than fifteen minutes at the beginning of the sleep period and are most likely to arise during the sleep transition or light sleep.

Rhythmic movement disorder can become a concern if movements occur frequently or in an older child. However, it rarely causes injury and usually does not have to be treated. The behavior is likely to go away over time. It may stop sooner if the parent brings the behavior to the child's attention and asks that it stop. If injury is occurring, behavioral therapy or benzodiazepine medication may help.

HEALTH PROBLEMS THAT CAN AFFECT SLEEP

In chapter 3, we talked about various health problems, from heart disease to allergies, that can fragment or disturb sleep. Following is information on some problems so linked to the sleep period that they are classified as sleep disorders.

Sleep-Related Headaches

Sleep-related headaches are migraine or cluster headaches. These headaches may awaken you during the middle of the night, or you may discover them in the morning. Sleep-related headaches begin during REM sleep when the blood vessels are more constricted.

Treatment is the same as for similar headaches during the day. See your doctor if the problem persists.

Sleep-Related Epilepsy

Many people with epilepsy have seizures during sleep and other sleep disturbances. Seizures may occur only during the day, only during sleep, or at both times. Sleep deprivation makes a seizure more likely.

A diagnosis of sleep-related epilepsy requires careful assessment of brain activity using an extensive number of sensors. The test is often purposefully scheduled when the person is suffering from sleep deprivation, as seizures are more likely to occur then.

Sleep-related epilepsy is treated with antiseizure medications. If the epilepsy is controlled during the day with medications, it will usually be controlled at night, too. If you have epilepsy, you should avoid sleep deprivation.

Sleep-Related Gastroesophageal Reflux

Gastroesophageal reflux—heartburn and acid regurgitation into the esophagus—is a sleep disorder that can contribute greatly to sleep problems. It's quite common. About one-third of Americans report at least occasional problems, and about 10 percent report chronic, ongoing problems. Symptoms are often worse after meals. Over time, the problem can lead to ulcers.

Lying down makes it easier for stomach fluids to wash up into the esophagus, which is why the problem often arises or significantly worsens during sleep. There are no ruder awakenings than those provoked by a burning sensation in your chest and the nasty taste of stomach acid in the back of your throat.

Treatment. Often the first step is to take antacids after the evening meal and just before going to sleep. Raise the head of your bed by placing wooden blocks under the headboard legs so that you sleep with your head higher than your feet. Gravity can then help keep the stomach fluids from washing up. Don't use pillows or bend your mattress—this practice may not help at all and may even make the condition worse. Although over-the-counter remedies such as Gaviscon are available, this problem warrants medical attention. So, as always, if you suffer from continued problems, see your doctor. There are prescription medications for combating the problem.

A combination of these approaches helped Victor, a middle-aged man who came to the Sleep Disorders Center complaining of disturbed nighttime sleep and daytime fatigue. Because he snored and was overweight, his doctor thought he might have sleep apnea, but an overnight laboratory test showed that his snoring was mild and his breathing was not disturbed. However, his sleep was quite fragmented. Multiple brief arousals during all stages of sleep increased Stage 1 sleep and somewhat reduced deep sleep. As we explored the possible causes for these arousals, we began to suspect that Victor was suffering from acid reflux at night. Follow-up testing using a probe to measure the acid in Victor's stomach at night confirmed that stomach acid was washing up into his esophagus during sleep.

Victor began using medication to reduce the amount of acid in his stomach. He also raised the head of his bed by about four inches to help keep stomach acids from washing into his esophagus. After only a couple of days, Victor called the office saying that his sleep was much improved and that he was feeling better during the day. Also, his success in treating his sleep disorder inspired him to watch his diet more carefully and lose a few extra pounds.

★ 11 ★

Consulting with a
Sleep Specialist

This book has been created to help you identify and treat many sleep problems yourself, but you may be interested in learning how a sleep specialist can help this process. If you suspect you have a sleep disorder or other medical problem, you certainly should seek professional help rather than trying to fix the problem yourself. This chapter will tell you what a sleep specialist is and what may happen if you work with one.

SLEEP SPECIALISTS AND SLEEP CENTERS

Sleep specialists are health practitioners with advanced degrees and clinical experience with sleep medicine. Most sleep specialists are physicians (M.D.), but some are osteopaths (D.O.), dentists (D.D.S.), or psychologists or other doctors (Ph.D.). Most have developed a primary specialty and have made sleep medicine a secondary area of specialty. For example, a physician may have a primary specialty in internal medicine, pulmonary medicine, neurology, or psychiatry and then have a secondary specialty in sleep medicine.

All sleep specialists must be certified by the American Board of Sleep Medicine. To obtain this certification, the clinician must have at least one year of practice in the field that has been supervised by a certified practitioner and then must pass a two-part examination of knowledge and practical skills. This process is arduous. No other certification is recognized for sleep specialists.

A sleep center is a unit that is dedicated to the evaluation and treatment of sleep disorders. Most centers are outpatient "clinics" that are affiliated with hospitals. Sleep centers formerly tended to be associated with large academic hospitals, but the growth of sleep medicine has resulted in sleep centers popping up even in smaller community hospitals. Typically the sleep center is located in a separate, quiet suite somewhere in the hospital or in a nearby office building. It is set up to provide sleepers with a comfortable, homelike environment.

If your primary care physician has an affiliation with a hospital that has a sleep center, choosing that center can facilitate communications between the sleep specialist and your usual doctor.

Each sleep center is headed by a doctor and may have other doctors on staff, or may consult as needed with doctors affiliated with the hospital. The center's staff may also include certified technicians who administer tests. Many sleep centers are also research facilities, making them the leading edge of discoveries in the field.

The American Sleep Disorders Association accredits sleep-disorders centers. If a center has been operating for a few years, it should be accredited by the association. You are more certain of receiving high-quality care at a center that has successfully passed the accreditation process. A current list of accredited centers is at the back of this book.

Consider your comfort level before using one of the portable recording services that come into your home to do an overnight study. They can be intrusive. (Do you want a stranger in your home watching you sleep?) Make sure the service is run by an accredited sleep center.

The Growth of Sleep Medicine

If you had a sleep problem in the 1950s and wanted to be seen by a sleep specialist, your family and friends, and even your doctor, would have had no idea what you were talking about. Little research existed in the area of sleep disorders, and few people in the country had clinical expertise in the field. Back then, people with sleep problems had no place to turn, and many endured their problem—and in some cases, unfair criticism and misunderstandings—with no hope for understanding or treatment.

Things began to change in the 1960s. The Association for the Psychophysiological Study of Sleep was formed as a professional organization for sleep researchers. In 1963 Dr. William Dement, a physician and sleep researcher from the University of Chicago, started a narcolepsy clinic at Stanford University. He and a colleague began to see people with daytime sleepiness. Their evaluations included daytime sleep testing, and they started offering medication treatments to their patients. Although this clinic later closed, it established an enduring model for the practice of sleep medicine that included office visits and specialized sleep recording in the diagnosis and treatment of sleep disorders.

The 1960s were also a rich time in other research related to sleep and sleep disorders. Benzodiazepine sleeping pills became available. The problem of sleep apnea was identified and became a focus of diagnosis and treatment. Methods of overnight sleep testing and daytime nap testing were improved.

In 1975 the Association of Sleep Disorders Centers was formed, with five members in the United States. This group later grew into the American Sleep Disorders Association (ASDA), which is the flagship organization in the field, offering professional membership, conferences, educational materials, and certification of sleep centers. The ASDA's work toward establishing credentials for clinical practitioners led to the birth of the American Board of Sleep Medicine, which currently certifies sleep specialists.

The growth of the field in the last two decades has been dramatic. As of fall 1996, there are 888 clinicians who are board certified in sleep medicine. In addition, 310 sleep-disorders clinics are accredited by the American Sleep Disorders Association—tremendous growth from the five centers that started it all. If you need help in the 1990s, you can turn to sleep specialists and sleep centers that have knowledge based on thousands of research studies and a wealth of experience.

Choosing a Sleep Specialist

Sleep specialists are available in most parts of the country. Here are some ways to find the specialist who is right for you.

- Ask your primary care physician for a referral to a specialist who has a solid reputation. If your doctor has a working relationship with the specialist, the effectiveness and ease with which they discuss your case may increase.
- Find a specialist in your area so you can return for follow-up visits if necessary.
- Consider the volume of patients that the specialist usually sees. Someone who sees many patients may have a broader range of experience than someone who sees very few. Ask if the doctor practices full-time in sleep medicine.
- Consider the type of patients that the specialist usually sees. For example, some sleep specialists treat only people with sleep-related breathing disorders such as sleep apnea, and some treat only people with insomnia. Other specialists will see people with any type of sleep problem. Make sure that the specialist is prepared to deal with your problem.
- Consider the terms of your health care coverage. Most private insurance carriers will cover a substantial portion of the cost of seeing a sleep specialist. Managed care insurers or health maintenance organizations may have in-network specialists or may cover a portion of your visit to an out-of-network specialist. Also, most sleep specialists take Medicare.
- Most sleep specialists work in sleep-disorders centers. If the center has been operating more than a few years, make sure it's accredited by the American Sleep Disorders Association.

THE CONSULTATION

When new patients call my office in Manhattan, a common question is, If I come in to see you, what will you do? Here's what you can expect during your first visit to a sleep specialist, which is called the consultation.

The Interview

The doctor will first interview you about your sleep problems and sleep habits. Most sleep specialists will take considerable time to learn about you. Our consultations at the Institute, while sometimes around thirty minutes long, have been known to extend beyond two hours for complicated cases.

Once your consultation gets under way, it's common for the doctor to say, "Tell me what brings you to consult with a sleep specialist at this time." You then have an opportunity to describe the problem that you're having and the extent to which it affects your life.

No matter how thoroughly you explain your problem, be prepared for the doctor to ask you several detailed questions about your sleep. The doctor will want to know the times you get into bed, turn out the lights, and fall asleep; how many times you wake up each night; and how long you stay awake. And it's important to know the time of your final awakening, the time you get out of bed, and if you feel sleepy or nap after rising. Don't be surprised if the doctor asks questions about your habits or behavior during the night or day or about your thoughts and feelings. For example, people with insomnia are commonly asked, "What's on your mind when you're awake during the night, and what kinds of things do you do when you can't sleep?"

It's really helpful if you can tell the doctor when your symptoms are at their worst and any times that they seem to improve, especially if you have an idea of why the severity changes. For example, someone who snores might notice that his snoring is worst when he sleeps on his back or during allergy season or when he's gained a few pounds.

Once you've had an opportunity to talk about the specifics of your problem with the doctor, you may be asked a series of questions designed to unearth other existing sleep problems. For example, a person with insomnia may be asked about symptoms of snoring, sleep apnea, narcolepsy, or parasomnia. Such questions help the doctor be very thorough and complete in making your diagnosis. It's also quite common for the doctor to ask about your past sleep experiences: "Any sleep problems as a child or young adult?"

In the next phase of the interview the doctor is likely to ask whether you have any medical or psychiatric conditions that may affect your sleep. This phase will include questions about your use of medications and other substances such as caffeine, alcohol, and nicotine. The doctor will also want to know if you've ever suffered from depression, anxiety, or other emotional disturbance, since these may contribute to some types of sleep problems.

Near the end of the interview the doctor may ask you about your family history because this information can sometimes help guide diagnosis or treatment. Finally, the doctor may ask you about treatments that you have tried before and how effective they were. If you've tried many treatments, you might want to write them down before going in for your visit. If the treatments have involved medicines, write them down, too. Be sure to note any positive responses as well as any adverse reactions to any medicines you have taken.

Physical Examination

Most consultations with a sleep specialist involve a brief physical examination to make sure no physical or medical conditions are contributing to your sleep problem. If you're a snorer, the doctor may carefully examine your airway. Since sexual problems do not interrelate with sleep problems, the examination usually does not include a genital or breast exam. If you have recently had a physical examination performed by your primary care physician, take a copy of the report along to your consultation.

If the doctor suspects that a medical or psychiatric problem may be a contributing factor in your sleep problem, you may be asked to have tests. For example, you may need an electrocardiogram (EKG) to monitor your heart, a chest X ray, or blood tests. If the doctor suspects sleep apnea, he or she may also ask for special imaging studies of your airway. If a psychiatric problem is suspected, the sleep specialist might suggest that you speak with a psychiatrist or psychologist, or undergo some psychological testing, to determine the extent of the problem and the need for treatment.

Sleep Log

It's quite common to be asked to complete a sleep log either before the consultation visit or immediately afterwards. As you know from chapter 4, a sleep log is one of the most valuable tools for understanding sleep habits and needs, and it will help the doctor complete the diagnostic examination and make appropriate treatment recommendations.

If the specialist doesn't send you a sleep log before the consultation, you can use the one in this book and take it to your appointment. Either way, complete your sleep log as accurately as you can and write down anything that might be related to your sleep habits or patterns. For example, write down if you've used caffeine, alcohol, or nicotine or if you've recently traveled outside of your home time zone. Try to give the specialist as clear a picture of your sleep patterns as possible from the very first visit.

SLEEP TESTING

Many people, though not all, who are seen for consultation by a sleep specialist are asked to return to the center for an overnight sleep study or a daytime nap study. These tests are sometimes required for an accurate diagnosis and appropriate treatment plan. After you complete your consultation, one of the three following plans will be selected:

- **Overnight sleep study not recommended.** A treatment plan will probably be established without sleep testing.
- **Overnight sleep study recommended.** An overnight study must be done before a treatment can be started.
- **Overnight sleep study deferred.** The doctor may prefer to do the overnight study later. Perhaps you just started taking a new medication or just returned from travel abroad or are recovering from an illness. Or perhaps the doctor wants to try a treatment and then bring you back for an overnight test only if that treatment fails to improve your sleep.

Overnight Sleep Studies

Although an overnight sleep test is a medical test, for most people it is a novel and interesting experience. Believe or not, despite the common concern that "I won't be able to sleep if someone is monitoring me," almost everyone sleeps enough so that the doctor can interpret the test. One of the reasons that people sleep so well is that many sleep centers have bedrooms that are cozy and homey. At the very least, the test rooms are usually far removed from the hustle and bustle of the hospital and tend to be much quieter and more comfortable than a typical hospital bedroom.

Overnight sleep studies, also known as *nocturnal polysomnography,* require that you sleep while equipment monitors and records your brain activity, muscle activity, heart rate, breathing, and blood oxygen saturation. All of the tests are painless. Recording devices are placed only on the surfaces of the skin. Small electrodes (sensors) are applied to your scalp, face, chest, and lower legs for recording your sleep patterns. Airflow is usually measured with a small device that rests just below your nose, and your effort to breathe is measured with flexible belts that encircle your trunk at the chest and abdomen. Heart rate is measured with a sensor that's placed just over the heart; for women, the sensor is usually placed just underneath the breast. A finger probe uses a light to detect how much oxygen is in your blood. Some people, especially those with sensitive skin, may experience some irritation from the paste or tape used to apply the sensors or from the cleansing solutions for removing them. Otherwise, there should be no discomfort. Usually, the recording equipment is in another room so that the technician can observe the equipment without disturbing you. You may be observed during sleep with a closed-circuit TV camera that works with low light.

You prepare for an overnight sleep study pretty much like you'd prepare for an overnight trip to a friend's house or a motel. Pack a small bag with all of the items that you would normally need for overnight, including pajamas, slippers, and robe. Keep in mind that you may be monitored by male and female technicians, so pack suitable sleepwear. Do not take any valuables with you. Most sleep centers supply soap, towels, bed linens, pillows, and blankets. However, if you want anything special from home that might make your overnight stay more comfortable (such as your favorite pillow), check with the doctor and see if you can take it for your overnight test. Since the test involves paste that will leave a residue in your hair, be sure to pack a good comb or brush and don't forget shampoo!

Most sleep centers also do not stock prescription medication, so be sure that you pack whatever medication you may need for the night. Ask the sleep specialist whether you should take your usual medication on the night of the study. Also, prior to your study you should not make any changes to your usual sleep schedule that you have not thoroughly discussed with the sleep specialist.

On the day of your study:

• Wash your skin and hair before you arrive at the laboratory. This improves the ability of the technicians to comfortably apply and remove recording sensors. Shampoo your hair and don't apply oil, gel, or conditioner.

- Arrive at the center at your scheduled time. You will probably be asked to arrive in the evening shortly before your bedtime. The technician will show you to your room, answer any questions that you may have, and then give you an opportunity to change into your pajamas. Then the technician will apply the recording electrodes, which takes between a half hour and an hour. Arriving on time will help the technician serve you better.

- Do not use alcohol or nonprescription drugs (pain killers, cold tablets, etc.) on the day of your overnight study. Speak to the sleep specialist regarding the use of any medication if you think that you need it on the day of your test.

- Do not drink coffee or consume other caffeinated beverages after noontime on the day of your study.

- Finish your dinner before seven P.M. on the evening of your study.

- Contact the sleep-center doctor if your health changes before you come in for your overnight test. For example, if you develop a cold or respiratory infection, the test may have to be rescheduled. Women who have severe premenstrual symptoms or menstrual cramps may need to reschedule if these problems threaten to interfere with sleep on the night of the study.

Many people sleep throughout the recording period of the study. Even those with insomnia sleep enough for the doctor to get an accurate impression of the problem. But don't be alarmed or embarrassed if you need to get up. The technicians are prepared to deal with requests to go to the bathroom or get a glass of water. Sometimes the technicians may interrupt you! They may need to enter your room to fix a faulty sensor or adjust your covers a bit so the doctor can see your breathing or other movements.

When you awaken in the morning, the technician usually makes short order of removing all of the recording sensors. You can then either leave the center right away or shower and dress there. The technicians usually do not provide any information about your sleep study, but the doctor may come in and give you a preliminary report. These reports are given after the sleep tracing has been reviewed briefly. Sometimes the doctor can start treatment right after a preliminary review, but because the sleep tracing takes time to score and analyze, more extensive reports have to wait.

In recent years, new technology has made it possible for overnight sleep testing to be done with portable recording equipment. Technicians are now able to go to the patient's home, hospital, or nursing home to perform a sleep study. Your doctor or the specialists who are affiliated with your health care plan might determine whether you should have an overnight sleep study done at home. You may be able to request the type of study that you prefer, depending on the services offered by the sleep center.

One final note. You should address all of your concerns with your sleep specialist before coming in for the overnight study. He or she will probably not be present when you arrive for the study, so if you have special needs, let them be known early. If a child or an elderly parent might need assistance during the night, don't hesitate to ask the doctor if you can remain nearby to provide comfort and assistance.

Nap Testing

Sometimes overnight sleep studies are followed by daytime nap studies. The most common of these studies is called the multiple sleep latency test, which is the standard test of daytime sleepiness. This test is often essential in diagnosing narcolepsy.

In a multiple sleep latency test, you are given several opportunities to nap during the day at ten A.M., noon, two P.M., four P.M., and possibly at six P.M. While wearing your street clothes, with shoes off, and with sensors applied to your face and scalp to record sleep, you lie in bed in a quiet, dark, and temperature-controlled room and are instructed to "lie quietly, keep your eyes closed, and try to fall asleep." The technician documents the amount of time that it takes you to fall asleep and the doctor can later interpret the findings.

The multiple sleep latency test is the best way that sleep specialists can determine your levels of sleepiness during the day. This information can be very important in determining your treatment plan. For example, if you have "mild" sleep apnea but are extremely sleepy during the day, the doctor may be more inclined to pursue treatment than if you were quite alert and functioning at a peak level all day.

Another daytime test is the maintenance of wakefulness test. This test is similar to the multiple sleep latency test, but this time you are instructed to remain awake rather than to fall asleep. This test can be important in documenting your capacity to stay awake and can help to document treatment success. It's sometimes critical in assessing whether treatment has helped people with high-risk jobs, such as truck drivers, pilots, or other transportation workers.

Not too long ago I was asked to meet with Mr. Smitty, a truck driver who routinely traveled a route between New York City and Alabama. Mr. Smitty worked for a New York–based trucking company, hauling fuels and fertilizers, and was referred to the Institute after he fell asleep behind the wheel of his truck and had a minor accident. Although he did no damage to his truck and injured no one, he ran over several barriers that had been placed in the road to warn of road construction ahead. If a crew member had been working, it could have been a disaster.

Mr. Smitty was seen for consultation, at which time I suspected that he had sleep apnea. An overnight sleep study confirmed the diagnosis, and a multiple sleep latency test revealed severe daytime sleepiness. Consequently, Mr. Smitty was given a paid leave of absence from his driving responsibilities at work while we began treatment with nasal continuous positive air pressure, a device that ensured that he had adequate airflow and oxygen despite his sleep apnea. Within a week we noted a major improvement in his nighttime sleep and breathing. However, a repeat multiple sleep latency test suggested that, while his sleepiness was greatly improved, he was still borderline. We waited a few more weeks while Mr. Smitty got more and more used to his device at night, and then we brought him back for testing with the maintenance of wakefulness test. To everyone's satisfaction, Mr. Smitty was able to remain awake and alert through the entire day of testing. This result gave us the satisfaction that he was adequately treated and gave his employers the confidence that they needed to return him to active duty on the road.

Reports

Overnight sleep study and daytime nap studies generate continuous recordings. For every second that you're being monitored, multiple channels of information are gathered. It takes a long time to analyze this wealth of information. A technician will need three to four hours to score an average overnight sleep recording, and then the sleep specialist will need additional time to review, analyze, and interpret the results. Consequently, the results of your sleep study may not become available for several days. After waiting several days, if you haven't received a call or been seen for a follow-up visit by the sleep specialist, call to find out when your test results can be expected.

Once your report becomes available, be sure that it's sent to your primary care doctor or to the doctor who sent you for sleep testing or to both. Some centers will also give you a copy.

FOLLOWING THROUGH

Once you've finished with sleep testing, you've really only begun on the road to treatment. Following the sleep test, you should have a clear idea from the sleep specialist of the treatment plan and who will conduct it. Sometimes treatment is done at the sleep center, sometimes it's started at the sleep center and then continued by your own doctor, and sometimes the sleep specialist will provide a treatment recommendation to your doctor who will carry out the treatment entirely. Whatever the case, you should be clear about the plan, its anticipated risks and benefits, and the steps you need to take.

Sometimes treatments are administered by allied health care professionals. A behavioral therapist may provide treatment for insufficient sleep, insomnia, circadian rhythm disorders, and so on. Or a respiratory therapist or home care agency may be called to dispense lifesaving equipment for continuous positive air pressure to a person with sleep apnea. These people will be acting on the recommendations of the sleep specialist to carry out a treatment plan.

Sometimes you will return to the sleep laboratory for tests to insure that the treatment has been effective. For example, a person who has severe sleep apnea and is treated with a combination of weight loss and surgery may be asked to return to the sleep center to ensure that the apnea has improved and that he is in good health.

Whatever treatment path you choose for your sleep problem, be sure to follow through with your doctor or the sleep specialist. A visit after being in treatment for a few months can be very important in shaping your long-term treatment plan and in keeping you comfortable with the way your treatment is progressing.

The most important person during the follow-up is, of course, you.

You need to follow the plan that you and the sleep specialist have formed. Whether your role is sticking to a new sleep schedule, taking prescribed medication, learning a relaxation technique, modifying your sleep behavior, or making changes in your lifestyle, you have a critical role. If all goes as it should, you will soon be getting the good nights of sleep that you deserve.

Directory of Sleep Centers

Following is a listing of sleep disorders centers that have been accredited by the American Sleep Disorders Association for the diagnosis and treatment of all types of sleep-related disorders. Accredited Member Laboratories, marked with an asterisk, treat only sleep-related breathing disorders. You can obtain a current listing and additional information from the American Sleep Disorders Association World Wide Web site at http://www.asda.org.

For information regarding Dr. Zammit's programs for treating sleep deprivation and other sleep disorders, please write to him at the Sleep Disorders Institute, 1090 Amsterdam Avenue, New York, NY 10025. You may also reach his private office by telephone at 914-646-1770.

ALABAMA

Brookwood Sleep Disorders Center
Brookwood Medical Center
2010 Brookwood Medical Center
  Drive
Birmingham, AL 35209
205-877-2486

Sleep Disorders Center of
  Alabama, Inc.
790 Montclair Road
Suite 200
Birmingham, AL 35213
205-599-1020

Sleep-Wake Disorders Center
University of Alabama at
 Birmingham
1713 6th Avenue South
CPM Building, Room 270
Birmingham, AL 35233-0018
205-934-7110

Sleep-Wake Disorders Center
Flowers Hospital
4370 West Main Street
PO Box 6907
Dothan, AL 36302
334-793-5000 x1685

Alabama North Regional Sleep
 Disorders Center
250 Chateau Drive
Suite 235
Huntsville, AL 35801
205-880-6451

Huntsville Hospital Sleep Disorders
 Center
101 Sivley Road
Huntsville, AL 35801
205-517-8553

Sleep Disorders Center
Mobile Infirmary Medical Center
PO Box 2144
Mobile, AL 36652
334-431-5559

Southeast Regional Center for
 Sleep/Wake Disorders
Springhill Memorial Hospital
3719 Dauphin Street
Mobile, AL 36608
334-460-5319

USA Knollwood Sleep Disorders
 Center
University of South Alabama

Knollwood Park Hospital
5600 Girby Road
Mobile, AL 36693-3398
334-660-5757

Baptist Sleep Disorders Center
Baptist Medical Center
2105 East South Boulevard
Montgomery, AL 36116-2498
334-286-3252

Tuscaloosa Clinic Sleep Lab*
701 University Boulevard East
Tuscaloosa, AL 35401
205-349-4043

ALASKA

Sleep Disorders Center
Providence Alaska Medical Center
3200 Providence Drive
PO Box 196604
Anchorage, AK 99519-6604
907-261-3650

ARIZONA

Samaritan Regional Sleep Disorders
 Program
Desert Samaritan Medical Center
1400 South Dobson Road
Mesa, AZ 85202
602-835-3620

Samaritan Regional
 Sleep Disorders Program
Good Samaritan Regional Medical
 Center
1111 East McDowell Road
Phoenix, AZ 85006
602-239-5815

Sleep Disorders Center at Scottsdale
 Memorial Hospital

Scottdale Memorial Hospital–North
10450 North 92nd Street
Scottsdale, AZ 85261-9930
602-860-3200

Sleep Disorder Center
University of Arizona
1501 North Campbell Avenue
Tucson, AZ 85724
520-694-6112

ARKANSAS

Sleep Disorder Center
Washington Regional Medical
    Center
1125 North College Avenue
Fayetteville, AR 72703
501-442-1272

Pediatric Sleep Disorders
Arkansas Children's Hospital
800 Marshall Street
Little Rock, AR 72202-3591
501-320-1893

Sleep Disorders Center
Baptist Medical Center
9601 I-630, Exit 7
Little Rock, AR 72205-7299
501-227-1902

CALIFORNIA

WestMed Sleep Disorders Center
1101 South Anaheim Boulevard
Anaheim, CA 92805
714-491-1159

Mercy Sleep Laboratory*
Mercy San Juan Hospital
6501 Coyle Avenue

Carmichael, CA 95608
916-966-5552

Palomar Medical Center Sleep
    Disorders Lab*
Palomar Medical Center
555 East Valley Parkway
Escondido, CA 92025
619-739-3457

Sleep Disorders Institute
St. Jude Medical Center
100 East Valencia Mesa Drive
Suite 308
Fullerton, CA 92635
714-992-3981

Glendale Adventist Medical Center
    Sleep Disorders Center
Glendale Adventist Medical Center
1509 Wilson Terrace
Glendale, CA 91206
818-409-8323

Sleep Disorders Center
Scripps Clinic and Research
    Foundation
10666 North Torrey Pines Road
La Jolla, CA 92037
619-554-8087

Sleep Disorders Center
Grossmont Hospital
PO Box 158
La Mesa, CA 91944-0158
619-644-4488

Loma Linda Sleep Disorder Center
Loma Linda University Medical
    Center
11234 Anderson Street
Loma Linda, CA 92354
909-478-8380

Memorial Sleep Disorders Center
Long Beach Memorial Medical
 Center
2801 Atlantic Avenue
PO Box 1428
Long Beach, CA 90801-1428
310-933-2091 or 310-426-1816

Sleep Disorders Center
Cedars-Sinai Medical Center
8700 Beverly Boulevard
Los Angeles, CA 90048-1869
310-855-2405

UCLA Sleep Disorders Center
710 Westwood Plaza
Los Angeles, CA 90095
310-206-8005

Sleep Disorders Center
Hoag Memorial Hospital
 Presbyterian
301 Newport Boulevard
PO Box 6100
Newport Beach, CA 92658-6100
714-760-2070

Sleep Evaluation Center
Northridge Hospital Medical Center
18300 Roscoe Boulevard
Northridge, CA 91328
818-885-5344

California Center for Sleep
 Disorders
3012 Summit Street
5th Floor, South Building
Oakland, CA 94609
510-834-8333

St. Joseph Hospital Sleep Disorders
 Center
1310 West Stewart Drive
Suite 403

Orange, CA 92668
714-771-8950

University of California, Irvine
Sleep Disorders Center
101 City Drive, Route 23
Orange, CA 92668
714-456-5105

Sleep Disorders Center
Huntington Memorial Hospital
100 West California Boulevard
PO Box 7013
Pasadena, CA 91109-7013
818-397-3061

Sleep Disorders Center
Doctors Hospital–Pinole
2151 Appian Way
Pinole, CA 94564-2578
510-741-2525 and 800-640-9440

Pomona Valley Hospital Medical
 Center
Sleep Disorders Center
1798 North Garey Avenue
Pomona, CA 91767
909-865-9587

The Center for Sleep Apnea*
Redding Specialty Hospital
2801 Eureka Way
Redding, CA 96002
916-245-4187

Sleep Disorders Center
Sequoia Hospital
170 Alameda de las Pulgas
Redwood City, CA 94062-2799
415-367-5137

Sleep Disorders Center at Riverside
Riverside Community Hospital
4445 Magnolia, E1

Riverside, CA 92501
909-788-3377

Sutter Sleep Disorders Center
650 Howe Avenue
Suite 910
Sacramento, CA 95825
916-646-3300

Mercy Sleep Disorders Center
Mercy HealthCare San Diego
4077 Fifth Avenue
San Diego, CA 92103-2180
619-260-7378

San Diego Sleep Disorders Center
1842 Third Avenue
San Diego, CA 92101
619-235-0248

UCSF/Mt. Zion Sleep Disorders
  Center
University of California, San
  Francisco
1600 Divisadero Street
San Francisco, CA 94115
415-885-7886

Sleep Disorders Center
San Jose Medical Center
675 East Santa Clara Street
San Jose, CA 95112
408-993-7005

The Sleep Disorders of Santa
  Barbara
2410 Fletcher Avenue
Suite 201
Santa Barbara, CA 93105
805-898-8845

Sleep Disorders Clinic
Stanford University

401 Quarry Road
Stanford, CA 94305
415-723-6601

Southern California Sleep Apnea
  Center*
Lombard Medical Group
2230 Lynn Road
Thousand Oaks, CA 91360
805-495-1066

Torrance Memorial Medical Center
Sleep Disorders Center
3330 West Lomita Boulevard
Torrance, CA 90505
310-517-4617

Sleep Disorders Laboratory*
Kaweah Delta District Hospital
400 West Mineral King Avenue
Visalia, CA 93291
209-625-7338

West Hills Sleep Disorders
  Center
23101 Sherman Place
Suite 108
West Hills, CA 91307
818-715-0096

Sleep Disorders Center
Woodland Memorial Hospital
1325 Cottonwood Street
Woodland, CA 95695
916-668-2695

COLORADO

National Jewish/University of
  Colorado Sleep Center
1400 Jackson Street, A200
Denver, CO 80206
303-398-1523

Sleep Center of Southern
 Colorado
Parkview Episcopal Medical Center
400 West Sixteenth Street
Pueblo, CO 81003
719-584-4659

CONNECTICUT

Danbury Hospital Sleep Disorders
 Center
Danbury Hospital
24 Hospital Avenue
Danbury, CT 06810
203-731-8033

New Haven Sleep Disorders Center
100 York Street
University Towers
New Haven, CT 06511
203-776-9578

Gaylord-Yale Sleep Disorders
 Laboratory*
Gaylord Hospital
Gaylord Farms Road
Wallingford, CT 06492
203-284-2853

DELAWARE

No Accredited Member Centers

DISTRICT OF COLUMBIA

Sibley, Memorial Hospital Sleep
 Disorders Center
5255 Loughboro Road Northwest
Washington, DC 20016
202-364-7676

Sleep Disorders Center
Georgetown University Hospital
3800 Reservoir Road, Northwest

Washington, DC 20007-2197
202-784-3610

FLORIDA

Boca Raton Sleep Disorders Center
899 Meadows Road
Suite 101
Boca Raton, FL 33486
407-750-9881

Sleep Disorder Laboratory*
Broward General Medical Center
1600 South Andrews Avenue
Fort Lauderdale, FL 33316
954-355-5534

Center for Sleep Disordered
 Breathing*
PO Box 2982
Jacksonville, FL 32203
904-387-7300 x8743

Mayo Sleep Disorders Center
Mayo Clinic Jacksonville
4500 San Pablo Road
Jacksonville, FL 32224
904-953-7287

Watson Clinic Sleep Disorders
 Center
The Watson Clinic
1600 Lakeland Hills Boulevard
PO Box 95000
Lakeland, FL 33804-5000
941-680-7627

Atlantic Sleep Disorders Center
1401 South Apollo Boulevard
Melbourne, FL 32901
407-952-5191

Sleep Disorders Center
Miami Children's Hospital

6125 Southwest 31st Street
Miami, FL 33155
305-662-8330

University of Miami School
 of Medicine, JMH and VA
 Medical Center Sleep Disorders
 Center
Department of Neurology (D4-5)
PO Box 016960
Miami, FL 33101
305-324-3371

Sleep Disorders Center
Mt Sinai Medical Center
4300 Alton Road
Miami Beach, FL 33140
305-674-2613

Florida Hospital Sleep Disorders
 Center
601 East Rollins Avenue
Orlando, FL 32803
407-897-1558

Health First Sleep Disorders Center
Palm Bay Community Hospital
1425 Malabar Road Northeast
Suite 255
Palm Bay, FL 32907
407-728-5387

Sleep Disorders Center
Sarasota Memorial Hospital
1700 South Tamiami Trail
Sarasota, FL 34239
941-917-2525

St. Petersburg Sleep Disorders
 Center
2525 Pasadena Avenue South
Suite S
St. Petersburg, FL 33707

813-360-0853 and 800-242-3244
 (in Florida)

Laboratory for Sleep Related
 Breathing Disorders*
University Community Hospital
3100 East Fletcher Avenue
Tampa, FL 33613
813-979-7410 x7410

GEORGIA

Atlanta Center for Sleep Disorders
303 Parkway
Box 44
Atlanta, GA 30312
404-265-3722

Sleep Disorders Center
Northside Hospital
1000 Johnson Ferry Road
Atlanta, GA 30342
404-851-8135

Sleep Disorders Center of Georgia
5505 Peachtree Dunwoody Road
Suite 370
Atlanta, GA 30342
404-257-0080

Sleep Disorders Center
Promina Kennestone Hospital
677 Church Street
Marietta, GA 30060
770-793-5353

Department of Sleep Disorders
 Medicine
Candler Hospital
5353 Reynolds Street
Savannah, GA 31405
912-692-6531

Savannah Sleep Disorders Center
Saint Joseph's Hospital
#6 St. Joseph's Professional Plaza
11706 Mercy Boulevard
Savannah, GA 31419
912-927-5141

Sleep Disorders Center
Memorial Medical Center, Inc.
4700 Waters Avenue
Savannah, GA 31403
912-350-8327

HAWAII

Pulmonary Sleep Disorders Center*
Kuakini Medical Center
347 North Kuakini Street
Honolulu, HI 96817
808-547-9119

Sleep Disorders Center of the Pacific
Straub Clinic & Hospital
888 South King Street
Honolulu, HI 96813
808-522-4448

IDAHO

Idaho Sleep Disorders Laboratory
St. Luke's Regional Medical Center
190 East Bannock Street
Boise, ID 83712
208-381-2440

ILLINOIS

Neurological Testing Center's
  Sleep Disorders Center
Northwestern Memorial Hospital
303 East Superior, Passavant 1044
Chicago, IL 60611
312-908-8120

Sleep Disorders Center
The University of Chicago
  Hospitals
5841 South Maryland
MC2091
Chicago, IL 60637
312-702-1782

Sleep Disorder Service and Research
  Center
Rush-Presbyterian-St. Luke's
1653 West Congress Parkway
Chicago, IL 60612
312-942-5440

Sleep Disorders Center
Evanston Hospital
2650 Ridge Avenue
Evanston, IL 60201
847-570-2567

C. Duane Morgan Sleep Disorders
  Center
Methodist Medical Center
  of Illinois
221 Northeast Glen Oak Avenue
Peoria, IL 61636
309-672-4966

SIU School of Medicine/Memorial
  Medical Center
Sleep Disorders Center
Memorial Medical Center
800 North Rutledge
Springfield, IL 62781
217-788-4269

Carle Regional Sleep Disorders
  Center
Carle Foundation Hospital
611 West Park Street
Urbana, IL 61801-2595
217-383-3364

INDIANA

St. Mary's Sleep Disorders Center*
St. Mary's Medical Center
3700 Washington Avenue
Evansville, IN 47750
812-479-4960

St. Joseph Sleep Disorders Center
St. Joseph Medical Center
700 Broadway
Fort Wayne, IN 46802
219-425-3552

Sleep Wake Disorders Center
Winona Memorial Hospital
3232 North Meridian Street
Indianapolis, IN 46208
317-927-2100

Sleep/Wake Disorders Center
Community Hospitals of
Indianapolis
1500 North Ritter Avenue
Indianapolis, IN 46219
317-355-4275

Sleep Alertness Center
Lafayette Home Hospital
2400 South Street
Lafayette, IN 47904
317-447-6811 x2840

Sleep Disorders Center
Good Samaritan Hospital
520 South 7th Street
Vincennes, IN 47591
812-885-3877

IOWA

Sleep Disorders Center
Genesis Medical Center

1401 West Central Park
Davenport, IA 52804
319-383-1966

Sleep Disorders Center
The Department of Neurology
The University of Iowa Hospitals
and Clinics
Iowa City, IA 52242
319-356-3813

KANSAS

Sleep Disorders Center
St. Francis Hospital and Medical
Center
1700 Southwest 7th Street
Topeka, KS 66606-1690
913-295-7900

Sleep Disorders Center
Wesley Medical Center
550 North Hillside
Wichita, KS 67214-4976
316-688-2663

KENTUCKY

Sleep Diagnostics Lab*
Greenview Regional Medical Center
1801 Ashley Circle
Bowling Green, KY 42101
502-793-2172

Sleep Lab*
The Medical Center at Bowling
Green
250 Park Street
PO Box 90010
Bowling Green, KY 42101-9010
502-745-1024

The Sleep Disorder Center of
St. Luke Hospital
St. Luke's Hospital, Inc.
85 North Grand Avenue
Fort Thomas, KY 41075
606-572-3535

Sleep Apnea Center*
Columbia Hospital of Lexington
310 South Limestone
Lexington, KY 40508
606-252-6612 x7331

Sleep Disorders Center
St. Joseph's Hospital
One St. Joseph's Drive
Lexington, KY 40504
606-278-0444

Sleep Disorders Center
Columbia Audubon Hospital
One Audubon Plaza Drive
Louisville, KY 40217
502-636-7459

Sleep Disorders Center
University of Louisville Hospital
530 South Jackson Street
Louisville, KY 40202
502-562-3792

Regional Medical Center Lab for
Sleep-Related Breathing Disorders*
900 Hospital Drive
Madisonville, KY 42431
502-825-5918

LOUISIANA

Mercy + Baptist Sleep Disorders
Center
2700 Napoleon Avenue
New Orleans, LA 70115
504-896-5439

Tulane Sleep Disorders Center
1415 Tulane Avenue
New Orleans, LA 70112
504-588-5231

LSU Sleep Disorders Center
Louisiana State University Medical
Center
PO Box 33932
Shreveport, LA 71130-3932
318-675-5365

The Neurology and Sleep Clinic
2205 East 70th Street
Shreveport, LA 71105
318-797-1585

MAINE

Maine Sleep Apnea Institute*
Maine Medical Center
22 Bramhall Street
Portland, ME 04102
207-871-2279

MARYLAND

Maryland Sleep Disorders Center, Inc.
Ruxton Towers, Suite 211
8415 Bellona Lane
Baltimore, MD 21204
410-494-9773

The Johns Hopkins Sleep Disorders
Center
Asthma and Allergy Building,
Room 4B50
Johns Hopkins Bayview Medical
Center
5501 Hopkins Bayview Circle
Baltimore, MD 21224
410-550-0571

Frederick Sleep Disorders Center
Frederick Memorial Hospital
400 West 7th Street
Frederick, MD 21701
301-698-3802

Shady Grove Sleep Disorders Center
14915 Broschart Road
Suite 102
Rockville, MD 20850
301-251-5905

Washington Adventist Sleep
  Disorders Center
7525 Carroll Avenue
Takoma Park, MD 20912
301-891-2594

MASSACHUSETTS

Sleep Disorders Center
Beth Israel Hospital
330 Brookline Avenue KS430
Boston, MA 02215
617-667-3237

Sleep Disorders Center
Lahey-Hitchcock Clinic
41 Mall Road
Burlington, MA 01805
617-273-8251

Sleep Disorders Institute of Central
  New England
St. Vincent Hospital
25 Winthrop Street
Worcester, MA 01604
508-798-6212

MICHIGAN

Sleep/Wake Disorders
  Laboratory (127B)

VA Medical Center
4646 John R.
Allen Park, MI 48202
313-576-1000 x3663 or 3662

Sleep Disorder
St. Joseph Mercy Hospital
PO Box 995
Ann Arbor, MI 48106
313-712-4651

Sleep Disorders Center
University of Michigan Hospital
1500 East Medical Center Drive
Med Inn C433, Box 0842
Ann Arbor, MI 48109-0115
313-936-9068

Sleep Disorders Clinic
Bay Medical Center
1900 Columbus Avenue
Bay City, MI 48708
517-894-3332

Sleep Disorders Center
Henry Ford Hospital
2921 West Grand Boulevard
Detroit, MI 48202
313-972-1800

Sleep Disorders Center
Butterworth Hospital
100 Michigan Street Northeast
Grand Rapids, MI 49503
616-732-3759

Sleep Disorders Center
W.A. Foote Memorial
  Hospital, Inc.
205 North East Avenue
Jackson, MI 49201
517-788-4750

Borgess Sleep Disorders Center
Borgess Medical Center
1521 Gull Road
Kalamazoo, MI 49001
Sue Cammarata, M.D.
616-226-7081

Michigan Capital Healthcare
Sleep/Wake Center
2025 South Washington Avenue
Suite 300
Lansing, MI 48910-0817
517-334-2510

Sparrow Sleep Center
Sparrow Hospital
1215 East Michigan Avenue
PO Box 30480
Lansing, MI 48909-7980
517-483-2946

Sleep Disorders Center
Oakwood Downriver Medical
    Center
25750 West Outer Drive
Lincoln Park, MI 48146-1599
313-382-6165

Sleep & Respiratory Associates of
    Michigan
28200 Franklin Road
Southfield, MI 48034
810-350-2722

Munson Sleep Disorders Center
Munson Medical Center
1105 6th Street
MPB Suite 307
Traverse City, MI 49684-2386
800-358-9641 or 616-935-6600

Sleep Disorders Institute
44199 Dequindre
Suite 311

Troy, MI 48098
810-879-0707

MINNESOTA

Duluth Regional Sleep Disorders
    Center
St. Mary's Medical Center
407 East Third Street
Duluth, MN 55805
612-347-6288

Minnesota Regional Sleep Disorders
    Center
Hennepin County Medical Center
701 Park Avenue South
Minneapolis, MN 55415
612-347-6288

Sleep Disorders Center
Abbott Northwestern Hospital
800 East 28th Street at Chicago
    Avenue
Minneapolis, MN 55407
612-863-4516

Mayo Sleep Disorders Center
Mayo Clinic
200 First Street Southwest
Rochester, MN 55407
507-266-8900

Sleep Disorders Center
Methodist Hospital
6500 Excelsior Boulevard
St. Louis Park, MN 55426
612-993-6083

St. Joseph's Sleep Diagnostic Center
St. Joseph's Hospital
69 West Exchange Street
St. Paul, MN 55102
612-232-3682

MISSISSIPPI

Sleep Disorders Center
Memorial Hospital at Gulfport
PO Box 1810
Gulfport, MS 39501
601-865-3152

Sleep Disorders Center
Forrest General Hospital
PO Box 16389
6051 Highway 49
Hattiesburg, MS 39404
601-288-4790 or 800-280-8520

Sleep Disorders Center
University of Mississippi Medical
  Center
2500 North State Street
Jackson, MS 39216-4505
601-984-4820

MISSOURI

Sleep Medicine and Research
  Center
St. Luke's Hospital
232 South Woods Mill Road
Chesterfield, MO 63017
314-205-6030

University of Missouri Sleep
  Disorders Center
M-741 Neurology
University Hospital
  and Clinics
One Hospital Drive
Columbia, MO 65212
573-884-SLEEP or
  800-ADD-SLEEP

Sleep Disorders Center
St. Luke's Hospital
4400 Wornall Road

Kansas City, MO 54111
816-932-3207

Sleep Disorders Center
Research Medical Center
2316 East Meyer Boulevard
Kansas City, MO 64132-1199
816-276-4334

Cox Regional Sleep Disorders Center
3800 South National Avenue
Suite LL 150
Springfield, MO 65807
417-269-5575

Sleep Disorders & Research Center
Deaconess Medical Center
6150 Oakland Avenue
St. Louis, MO 63139
314-768-3100

Sleep Disorders Center
St. Louis University Medical Center
1221 South Grand Boulevard
St. Louis, MO 63104
314-577-8705

MONTANA

No Accredited Member Centers

NEBRASKA

Great Plains Regional Sleep
  Physiology Center
Lincoln General Hospital
2300 South 16th Street
Lincoln, NE 68502
402-473-5338

Sleep Disorders Center
Clarkson Hospital
4350 Dewey Avenue
Omaha, NE 68105-1018
402-552-2286

Sleep Disorders Center
Methodist/Richard Young Hospital
2566 St. Mary's Avenue
Omaha, NE 68105
402-354-6305

NEVADA

Regional Center for Sleep
  Disorders
Sunrise Hospital and
  Medical Center
3186 South Maryland Parkway
Las Vegas, NV 89109
702-731-8365

The Sleep Clinic of Nevada
1012 East Sahara Avenue
Las Vegas, NV 89104
702-893-0020

Washoe Sleep Disorders Center and
  Sleep Laboratory
Washoe Professional Building and
  Wahoe Medical Center
75 Pringle Way, Suite 701
Reno, NV 89502
702-328-4700 or
  702-328-4701

NEW HAMPSHIRE

Sleep-Wake Disorders Center
Hampstead Hospital
East Road
Hampstead, NH 03841
603-329-5311 x240

Sleep Disorders Center
Dartmouth-Hitchcock Medical
  Center
One Medical Center Drive
Lebanon, NH 03756
603-650-7534

NEW JERSEY

Institute for Sleep/Wake Disorders
Hackensack University Medical
  Center
385 Prospect Avenue
Hackensack, NJ 07601
201-996-2992

Sleep Disorder Center
  of Morristown Memorial
  Hospital
95 Mount Kemble Avenue
2nd Floor, Thebaud Building
Morristown, NJ 07962
201-971-4567

Comprehensive Sleep Disorders
  Center
Robert Wood Johnson University
  Hospital/UMDNJ - Robert Wood
  Johnson Medical School
One Robert Wood Johnson Place
PO Box 2601
New Brunswick, NJ 08903
908-937-8683

Sleep Disorders Center
Newark Beth Israel
  Medical Center
201 Lyons Avenue
Newark, NJ 07112
201-926-7163

Mercer Medical Center Sleep
  Disorders Center
Mercer Medical Center
446 Bellevue Avenue
PO Box 1658
Trenton, NJ 08607
609-394-4167

Snoring and Sleep Apnea Center
Helene Fuld Medical Center
750 Brunswick Avenue

Trenton, NJ 08638
609-278-6990

NEW MEXICO

Lovelace Sleep Disorders
  Center
Lovelace Health Systems
2929 Coors Road NW
Suite 106
Albuquerque, NM 87102
505-839-2369

University Hospital Sleep
  Disorders Center
University of New Mexico
  Hospital
4775 Indian School Road Northeast
Suite 307
Albuquerque, NM 87110
505-272-6101

NEW YORK

Capital Region Sleep/Wake
  Disorders Center
St. Peter's Hospital and Albany
  Medical Center
25 Hackett Boulevard
Albany, NY 12208
518-436-9253

Sleep-Wake Disorders Center
Montefiore Medical Center
111 East 210th Street
Bronx, NY 10467
718-920-4841

St. Joseph's Hospital Sleep Disorders
  Center
St. Joseph's Hospital
555 East Market Street
Elmira, NY 14902
607-733-6541 x7008

Sleep Disorders Center
Winthrop–University Hospital
222 Station Plaza North
Mineola, NY 11501
516-663-3907

Sleep-Wake Disorders Center
Long Island Jewish Medical
  Center
270-05 76th Avenue
New Hyde Park, NY 11042
718-470-7058

Sleep Disorders Institute
St. Luke's–Roosevelt Hospital Center
1090 Amsterdam Avenue
New York, NY 10025
212-523-1700

The Sleep Disorders Center
Columbia Presbyterian Medical
  Center
161 Fort Washington Avenue
New York, NY 10032
212-305-1860

Sleep Disorders Center of Rochester
2110 Clinton Avenue South
Rochester, NY 14618
716-442-4141

Sleep Disorders Center
State University of New York at
  Stony Brook
University Hospital
MR 120 A
Stony Brook, NY 11794-7139
516-444-2916

The Sleep Center
Community General Hospital
Broad Road
Syracuse, NY 13215
315-492-5877

The Sleep Laboratory*
945 East Genesee Street
Suite 300
Syracuse, NY 13210
315-475-3379

Sleep-Wake Disorders Center
New York Hospital–Cornell Medical
  Center
21 Bloomingdale Road
White Plains, NY 10605
914-997-5751

NORTH CAROLINA

Sleep Medicine Center
  of Asheville
1091 Hendersonville Road
Asheville, NC 28803
704-277-7533

Sleep Center
University Hospital
PO Box 560727
Charlotte, NC 28256
704-548-5855

Sleep Disorders Center
The Moses H. Cone Memorial
  Hospital
1200 North Elm Street
Greensboro, NC 27401-1020
910-574-7406

Sleep Disorders Center
North Carolina Baptist Hospital
Bowman Gray School
  of Medicine
Medical Center Boulevard
Winston-Salem, NC 27157
910-716-5288

Summit Sleep Disorders Center
160 Charlois Boulevard

Winston-Salem, NC 27103
910-765-9431

NORTH DAKOTA

Sleep Disorders Center
MeritCare Hospital
720 4th Street North
Fargo, ND 58122
701-234-5673

OHIO

Sleep Disorders Center
Bethesda Oak Hospital
619 Oak Street
Cincinnati, OH 45206
513-569-6320

The Tri-State Sleep Disorders Center
1275 East Kemper Road
Cincinnati, OH 45246
513-671-3101

Sleep Disorders Center
Rainbow Babies Children's
  Hospital
Case Western Reserve University
11100 Euclid Avenue
Cleveland, OH 44106
216-844-1301

Sleep Disorders Center
The Cleveland Clinic Foundation
9500 Euclid Avenue
Desk S-83
Cleveland, OH 44195
216-444-8275

Sleep Disorders Center
The Ohio State University
  Medical Center
Rhodes Hall, S1039
410 West 10th Avenue

Columbus, OH 43210-1228
614-293-8296

The Center for Sleep & Wake
    Disorders
Miami Valley Hospital
One Wyoming Street
Suite G-200
Dayton, OH 45409
513-220-2515

Ohio Sleep Medicine and
    Neuroscience Institute
4975 Bradenton Avenue
Dublin, OH 43017
614-766-0773

Sleep Disorders Center
Kettering Medical Center
3535 Southern Boulevard
Kettering, OH 45429-1295
513-296-7805

Northwest Ohio Sleep
    Disorders Center
The Toledo Hospital
Harris-McIntosh Tower,
    Second Floor
2142 North Cove Boulevard
Toledo, OH 43606
419-471-5629

Sleep Disorders Center
St. Vincent Medical Center
2213 Cherry Street
Toledo, OH 43608-2691
419-321-4980

Sleep Disorders Center
Good Samaritan Medical Center
800 Forest Avenue
Zanesville, OH 43701
614-454-5855

OKLAHOMA

Sleep Disorders Center
of Oklahoma
Southwest Medical Center
of Oklahoma
4401 South Western Avenue
Oklahoma City, OK 73109
405-636-7700

OREGON

Sleep Disorders Center
Sacred Heart Medical Center
1255 Hilyard Street
PO Box 10905
Eugene, OR 97440
503-686-7224

Sleep Disorders Center
Rogue Valley Medical Center
2825 East Barnett Road
Medford, OR 97504
Eric Overland, M.D.
541-770-4320

Neurology, N-450
Legacy Good Samaritan Sleep
    Disorders Center
1015 Northwest 22nd Avenue
Portland, OR 97210
503-413-8170

Sleep Disorders Laboratory*
Providence Medical Center
4805 Northeast Glisan Street
Portland, OR 97213
503-215-6552

Salem Hospital Sleep Disorders
    Center
Salem Hospital
665 Winter Street Southeast
Salem, OR 97309-5014
503-370-5170

PENNSYLVANIA

Sleep Disorders Center
Abington Memorial Hospital
1200 Old York Road
2nd Floor Rorer Building
Abington, PA 19001
215-576-2226

Lehigh Valley Hospital Sleep
    Disorders Center
Lehigh Valley Hospital
Cedar Crest and I-78
PO Box 689
Allentown, PA 18105-1556
610-402-8532

Sleep Disorders Center
Lower Bucks Hospital
501 Bath Road
Bristol, PA 19007
215-785-9752

Sleep Disorders Center
    of Lancaster
Lancaster General Hospital
555 North Duke Street
Lancaster, PA 17604-3555
717-290-5910

Penn Center for Sleep Disorders
Hospital of the University of
    Pennsylvania
3400 Spruce Street
11 Gates West
Philadelphia, PA 19104
215-662-7772

Sleep Disorder Center
Thomas Jefferson University
1025 Walnut Street
Suite 316
Philadelphia, PA 19107
215-955-6175

Sleep Disorders Center
Medical College of Pennsylvania
    and Hahnemann
3200 Henry Avenue
Philadelphia, PA 19129
215-842-4250

Pulmonary Sleep Evaluation Center*
University of Pittsburgh Medical
    Center
Montefiore University Hospital
3459 Fifth Avenue, S639
Pittsburgh, PA 15213
412-692-2880

Sleep and Chronobiology Center
Western Psychiatric Institute
    and Clinic
3811 O'Hara Street
Pittsburgh, PA 15213-2593
412-624-2246

Sleep Disorders Center
Community Medical Center
1822 Mulberry Street
Scranton, PA 18510
717-969-8931

Sleep Disorders Center
Crozer-Chester Medical Center
One Medical Center Boulevard
Upland, PA 19013-3975
610-447-2689

Sleep Disorders Center
The Lankenau Hospital
100 Lancaster Avenue
Wynnewood, PA 19096
610-645-3400

RHODE ISLAND

Sleep Disorders Center
Rhode Island Hospital

593 Eddy Street, APC-301
Providence, RI 02903
401-444-4269

SOUTH CAROLINA

Roper Sleep/Wake Disorders Center
Roper Hospital
316 Calhoun Street
Charleston, SC 29401-1125
803-724-2246

Sleep Disorders Center of South
  Carolina
Baptist Medical Center
Taylor at Marion Streets
Columbia, SC 29220
803-771-5847

Sleep Disorders Center
Greenville Memorial Hospital
701 Grove Road
Greenville, SC 29605
864-455-8916

Children's Sleep Disorders Center*
Self Memorial Hospital
1325 Spring Street
Greenwood, SC 29646
803-227-4449 or 803-227-4489

Sleep Disorders Center
Spartanburg Regional Medical Center
101 East Wood Street
Spartanburg, SC 29303
803-560-6904

SOUTH DAKOTA

The Sleep Center
Rapid City Regional Hospital
353 Fairmont Boulevard
PO Box 6000
Rapid City, SD 57709
605-341-8037

Sleep Disorders Center
Sioux Valley Hospital
1100 South Euclid
Sioux Falls, SD 57117-5039
605-333-6302

TENNESSEE

Sleep Disorders Laboratory*
Regional Hospital of Jackson
367 Hospital Boulevard
Jackson, TN 38303
901-661-2148

Sleep Disorders Center
St. Mary's Medical Center
900 East Oak Hill Avenue
Knoxville, TN 37917-4556
423-545-6746

Sleep Disorders Center
Ft. Sanders Regional Medical
  Center
1901 West Clinch Avenue
Knoxville, TN 37916
423-541-1375

BMH Sleep Disorders Center
Baptist Memorial Hospital
899 Madison Avenue
Memphis, TN 38146
901-227-5337

Sleep Disorders Center
Methodist Hospital of Memphis
1265 Union Avenue
Memphis, TN 38104
901-726-REST

Sleep Disorders Center
Middle Tennessee Medical Center
400 North Highland Avenue
Murfreesboro, TN 37130
615-849-4811

Sleep Disorders Center
Centennial Medical Center
2300 Patterson Street
Nashville, TN 37203
615-342-1670

Sleep Disorders Center
Saint Thomas Hospital
PO Box 380
Nashville, TN 37202
615-222-2068

TEXAS

NWTH Sleep Disorders Center
Northwest Texas Hospital
PO Box 1110
Amarillo, TX 79175
806-354-1954

Sleep Disorders Center for Children
Children's Medical Center
  of Dallas
1935 Motor Street
Dallas, TX 75235
214-640-2793

Sleep Medicine Institute
Presbyterian Hospital of Dallas
8200 Walnut Hill Lane
Dallas, TX 75231
214-345-8563

Sleep Disorders Center
Columbia Medical Center West
1801 North Oregon
El Paso, TX 79902
915-521-1257

Sleep Disorders Center
Providence Memorial Hospital
2001 North Oregon
El Paso, TX 79902
915-577-6152

All Saints Sleep Disorders
  Diagnostic & Treatment Center
All Saints Episcopal Hospital
1400 8th Avenue
Fort Worth, TX 76104
817-927-6120

Sleep Disorders Center
Department of Psychiatry
Baylor College of Medicine and VA
  Medical Center
One Baylor Plaza
Houston, TX 77030
713-798-4886 or 713-794-7563

Sleep Disorders Center
Spring Branch Medical Center
8850 Long Point Road
Houston, TX 77055
713-973-6483

Sleep Disorder Center
Scott and White Clinic
2401 South 31st Street
Temple, TX 76508
817-724-2554

UTAH

Intermountain Sleep Disorders Center
LDS Hospital
325 8th Avenue
Salt Lake City, UT 84143
801-321-3617

University Health Sciences Center
Sleep Disorders Center
50 North Medical Drive
Salt Lake City, UT 84132
801-581-2016

VERMONT

No Accredited Member Centers

VIRGINIA

Fairfax Sleep Disorders Center
3289 Woodburn Road
Suite 360
Annandale, VA 22003
703-876-9871

Sleep Disorders Center for Adults
  and Children
Eastern Virginia Medical School
Sentara Norfolk General Hospital
600 Gresham Drive
Norfolk, VA 23507
804-668-3322

Sleep Disorders Center
Medical College of Virginia
PO Box 980710 - MCV
Richmond, VA 23298-0710
804-828-1490

Sleep Disorders Center
Community Hospital of Roanoke
  Valley
PO Box 12946
Roanoke, VA 24029
540-985-8526

WASHINGTON

Sleep Disorders Center for
  Southwest Washington
St. Peter Hospital
413 North Lilly Road
Olympia, WA 98506
360-493-7436

Richland Sleep Laboratory*
800 Swift Boulevard
Suite 260
Richland, WA 99352
509-946-4632

Providence Sleep Disorders
  Center
Jefferson Tower
Suite 203
1600 East Jefferson
Seattle, WA 98122
206-320-2575

Seattle Sleep Disorders Center
Swedish Medical Center/Ballard
PO Box 70707
Seattle, WA 98107-1507
206-781-6359

Sleep Disorders Center
Virginia Mason Medical Center
PO Box 1930 Mail Stop H10-SDC
925 Seneca Street
Seattle, WA 98111-1930
206-625-7180

Sleep Disorders Center
Sacred Heart Doctors Building
105 West Eighth Avenue
Suite 418
Spokane, WA 99204
509-455-4895

St. Clare Sleep Related Breathing
  Disorders Clinic*
St. Clare Hospital
11315 Bridgeport Way Southwest
Tacoma, WA 98499
206-581-6951

WEST VIRGINIA

Sleep Disorders Center
Charleston Area Medical Center
501 Morris Street
PO Box 1393
Charleston, WV 25325
304-348-7507

WISCONSIN

Regional Sleep Disorders Center
Appleton Medical Center
1818 North Meade Street
Appleton, WI 54911
414-738-6460

Luther/Midelfort Sleep
   Disorders Center
Luther Hospital/Midelfort
   Clinic
1221 Whipple Street
PO Box 4105
Eau Claire, WI 54702-4105
715-838-3165

St. Vincent Hospital Sleep
   Disorders Center
St. Vincent Hospital
PO Box 13508
Green Bay, WI 54307-3508
414-431-3041

Wisconsin Sleep Disorders
   Center
Gundersen Clinic, Ltd.
1836 South Avenue
La Crosse, WI 54601
608-782-7300 x2870

Comprehensive Sleep Disorders
   Center
B6/579 Clinical Science Center
University of Wisconsin Hospitals
   and Clinics
600 Highland Avenue
Madison, WI 53792
608-263-2387

Marshfield Sleep Disorders Center
Marshfield Clinic
1000 North Oak Avenue
Marshfield, WI 54449
715-387-5397

Milwaukee Regional Sleep Center
Columbia Hospital
2025 East Newport Avenue
Milwaukee, WI 53211
414-961-4650

St. Luke's Sleep Disorders Center
St. Luke's Medical Center
2900 West Oklahoma Avenue
Milwaukee, WI 53201-2901
414-649-6572

WYOMING

No Accredited Member Centers

Index